Atlas of Anatomy of Anal Canal

A Surgeon's Perspective

with

- **160+ illustrations**

Atlas of Anatomy of Anal Canal

A Surgeon's Perspective

with

• 160+ illustrations

Kamal Gupta MS FACS FAIS FACRSI
Consultant Colorectal Surgeon and Director
Karan Hospital, Jalandhar, India
Certified Trained Specialist in Laser Proctology, Berlin, Germany
Travelling Fellowship in Proctology, St. Mark's Hospital, London, UK
Fellow International Society of the University of Colon and Rectal Surgeons

Kushal Mital MS FACRSI
Consultant Surgeon and Director
Medicare Hospital, Thane and Govt CSMH, Kalwa, Thane, Mumbai

Niranjan Agarwal MS DNB FACRSI
Consultant, Laparoscopic and Colorectal Surgeon
Salasar Nursing Home, Bombay Hospital and Zen Multispecialty Hospital, Mumbai

CBSPD
CBS Publishers & Distributors Pvt Ltd
New Delhi • Bengaluru • Chennai • Kochi • Kolkata • Lucknow • Mumbai
Hyderabad • Jharkhand • Nagpur • Patna • Pune • Uttarakhand

Disclaimer

Science and technology are constantly changing fields. New research and experience broaden the scope of information and knowledge. The authors have tried their best in giving information available to them while preparing the material for this book. Although all efforts have been made to ensure optimum accuracy of the material, yet it is quite possible some errors might have been left uncorrected. The publisher, the printer and the authors will not be held responsible for any inadvertent errors, omissions or inaccuracies.

Atlas of
Anatomy of Anal Canal
A Surgeon's Perspective

with
• 160+ illustrations

ISBN: 978-93-5466-748-0

First Edition 2024

Published by Satish Kumar Jain and produced by Varun Jain for
CBS Publishers & Distributors Pvt Ltd
4819/XI Prahlad Street, 24 Ansari Road, Daryaganj, New Delhi 110 002, India
Ph: 011-23289259, 23266838 Website: www.cbspd.com
e-mail: delhi@cbspd.com

Corporate Office: 204 FIE, Industrial Area, Patparganj, Delhi 110 092, India
Ph: 011-49344934 Fax: 011-49344935
e-mail: publishing@cbspd.com; publicity@cbspd.com

Branches

- **Bengaluru:** Seema House 2975, 17th Cross, K.R. Road, Banasankari 2nd Stage, Bengaluru 560 070, Karnataka, India
  Ph: +91-80-26771678/79 Fax: +91-80-26771680 e-mail: bangalore@cbspd.com
- **Chennai:** 7, Subbaraya Street, Shenoy Nagar, Chennai 600 030, Tamil Nadu, India
  Ph: +91-44-26680620, 26681266 Fax: +91-44-42032115 e-mail: chennai@cbspd.com
- **Kochi:** 42/1325, 1326, Power House Road, Opposite KSEB, Power House, Ernakulum 682018, Kochi, Kerala, India
  Ph: +91-484-4059061–67 Fax: +91-484-4059065 e-mail: kochi@cbspd.com
- **Kolkata:** 147, Hind Ceramics Compound, 1st Floor, Nilgunj Road, Belghoria, Kolkata 700056, West Bengal, India
  Ph: +91-33-25330055/56 e-mail: kolkata@cbspd.com
- **Lucknow:** Basement, Khushuma Complex, 7 Meerabai Marg (behind Jawahar Bhawan), Lucknow 226001, UP, India
  Ph: +91-522-4000032 e-mail: tiwari.lucknow@cbspd.com
- **Mumbai:** PWD Shed, Gala No. 25/26, Ramchandra Bhatt Marg, Next JJ Hospital Gate No. 2, Opp. Union Bank of India, Noorbaug, Mumbai 400009, Maharashtra, India
  Ph: +91-22-66661880/89 e-mail: mumbai@cbspd.com

Representatives

- **Hyderabad** 0-9885175004
- **Jharkhand** 0-9811541605
- **Nagpur** 0-8692091830
- **Patna** 0-9334159340
- **Pune** 0-9664372571
- **Uttarakhand** 0-9716462459

Printed at Thomson Press India Ltd., Faridabad, Haryana, India

Preface

No knowledge can be more satisfactory to a man than that of his own frame, its parts, their functions and actions.

—Thomas Jefferson

At the very least, writing a book requires dedication, perseverance, and a passion for the subject. When my first book, *Lasers in Proctology*, was being published, I shared the anatomy chapters with Dr Indru Khubchandani for his review. Delighted to see the elaborative and descriptive anatomy illustrations, he suggested that I should come out with an atlas on the anatomy of the anal canal. His admiration of my previous work and a desire to create something valuable inspired me to pursue this project wholeheartedly.

Coming up with an atlas of a small part like the anal canal was not easy. After all, most of the textbooks complete the anatomy of this region in one and a half pages. Nevertheless, when I started thinking more and more about it, I realized there was so much to be discussed with the readers. For me, writing is a medium of communication with you all.

Some great surgeons and anatomists have worked hard to describe every structure of this tiny part known as *The Anal Canal*. Whether it was a description of the white line of Hilton by the great anatomist John Hilton popularly known as *Anatomical John*, the description of anal glands by Chiari, the correlation between anorectal abscesses and fistulas with anal glands or the pathways of spread of fistulas described by Eisenhammer or Sir Alan Park, the anatomy of sphincters and formation of anorectal ring by Milligan Morgan, anatomy of anal cushions by Thomson, the more I dug the literature, the more clarity started coming to my mind.

In this *Atlas of Anatomy of Anal Canal—A Surgeon's Perspective*, an attempt has been made to share the details of every structure present in the anal canal, the vascular supply, the lymphatic drainage, the innervation and the surgical significance. As surgeons, we know that operating and avoiding complications is impossible without understanding the surgical anatomy.

To make an atlas of this standard, I feel privileged to have Dr Kushal Mital and Dr Niranjan Aggarwal with me as coauthors. Both of them are great teachers and thoroughly understand the subject. The book has been divided into two parts, the second being *Atlas of Operative Proctology—A stepwise approach*. To thoroughly understand the operative procedures and avoid the most dreadful complications, recurrence and incontinence, the readers must go through the atlas of anatomy before going ahead with the operative atlas.

I want to take this opportunity to thank you all for appreciating my previous book, *Lasers in Proctology*, and making it a Bestselling Title.

As always, your suggestions are welcome. I promise to incorporate them in the next edition.

Kamal Gupta

"A beautiful rendition, a pictorial atlas with remarkably drawn skeletal, visceral, lymphovascular distribution and simple accompanying texts. You have introduced a unique volume to the readership of surgical and colorectal community students, practitioners and faculty".

Indru Khubchandani MD
Consultant Colorectal Surgeon, Pennsylvania

Acknowledgements

Chinese philosopher Lao Tzu once said, *The journey of a thousand miles begins with a single step*. I have been reading and listening to this proverb since my childhood. As a professional with a career expanding over three decades, I believe it does not matter how many steps one takes to complete a journey. To ensure success, one has to be determined, focused and obsessed.

I am not a strong advocate of the phrase, *I am a self-made man*, as I am not. There are so many helping hands in one's personal and professional life.

Walking alone and working in isolation is neither easy nor advisable. Having a companion with you can make even a long journey look short and worthwhile. My wife, Ruby, has been relentlessly there with me throughout my journey, always extending support at every step. As always, she has done an exceptional job reviewing the text from a learner's point of view and going through countless proofreadings. I want to thank her for her unwavering support, patience and constructive feedback.

A professional always flourishes with a mentor, and to find a friend in them is an icing on the cake. I take this opportunity to thank my mentor, Dr Kushal Mital and my dear friend, Dr Niranjan Aggarwal, for extending a helping hand while preparing illustrations for *the Atlas*. Finding a supportive team among these distinguished professionals makes this publication all the more special.

Writing a book requires much research. I want to thank my assistant, Dr Neeru Sahni, for conducting extensive research. The team has reviewed the expanse of literature published in the last century. I want to thank my office manager, Riya Sharma, for collecting the data, compiling it and helping me run my office smoothly while I was busy writing.

The credit for MRI images goes to the radiologist, Dr GS Bhola MD.

Having an idea in mind, creating rough drawings and converting them into elaborate illustrations is a professional job. I take this opportunity to thank Mr Brishank Pratap for his remarkable dedication in crafting illustrations for this book. Humouring medical professionals and delivering as per their expectations can be daunting for someone without a medical background. I can confidently say that he has done justice to the illustrations.

The credit for giving me an opportunity to interact and engage with young minds throughout this enlightening journey goes to Dr Suchitra Bindoria, the Director of IMMAST, Mumbai. She has been a pillar of support, and I am forever indebted to her for managing to take out time for me, even amidst her demanding commitments.

Lastly, I would like to thank CBS Publishers for publishing the Atlas and, through that, allowing the readers access to what I hope would offer a comprehensive understanding of the subject.

Kamal Gupta

Contents

CHAPTER 1

Anatomy of the Interior of the Anal Canal

The anal canal is the terminal part of the digestive tract between the rectum and the anus. Anteriorly the anal canal is separated from the vagina and the urethra by the perineal body. Posteriorly, it is separated from the coccyx by the anococcygeal ligament. Understanding the anatomy and function of the anal canal is essential in diagnosing and treating anorectal diseases.

ANAL CANAL

The anal canal runs anteroposteriorly and is enclosed by a strong muscular tube. It is entirely extraperitoneal (Fig. 1.1).

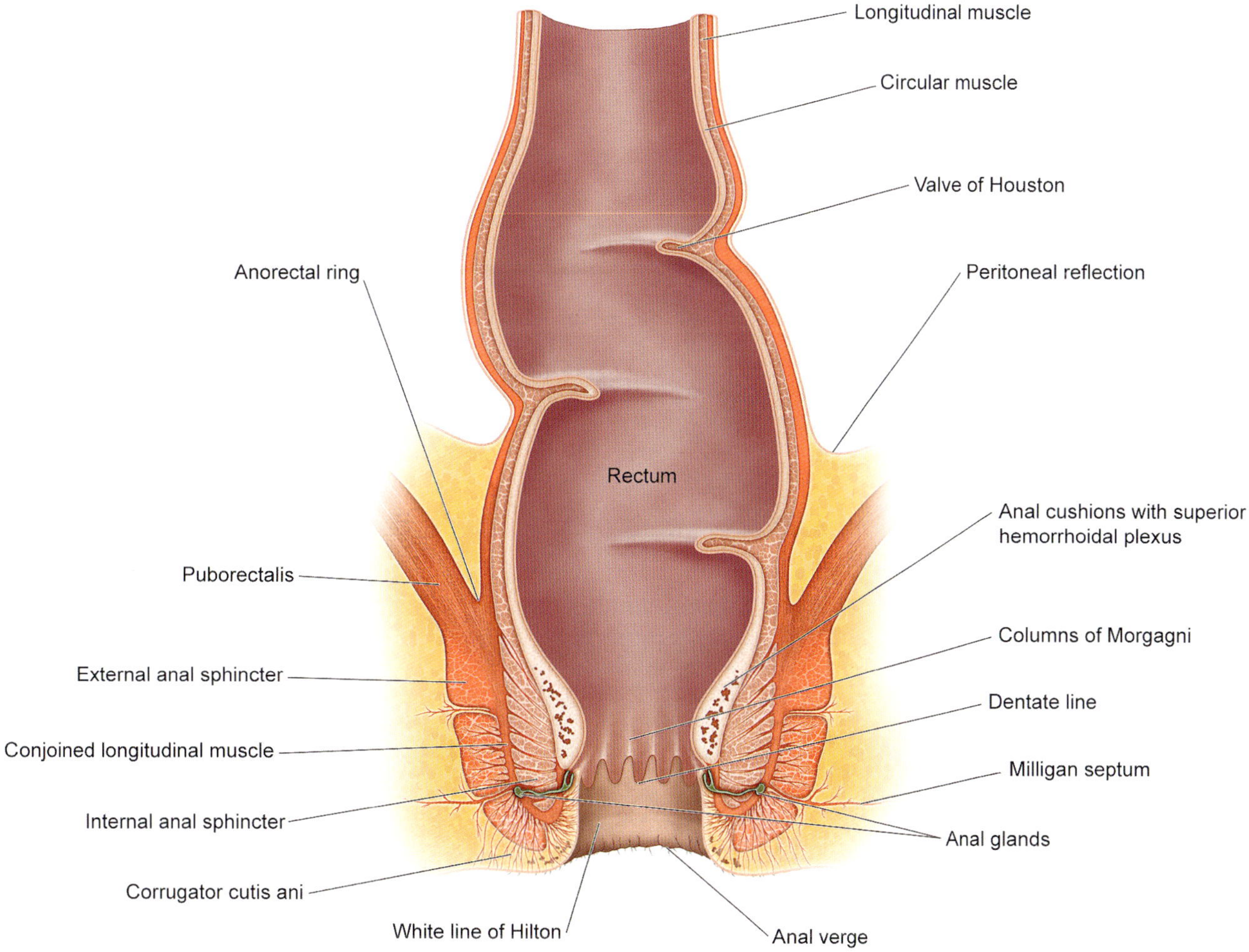

Fig. 1.1: Anal canal

The anal canal is described in two ways:

- **Anatomical anal canal**
  - 1.5–2.0 cm long
  - Extends from the anal verge to the dentate line
- **Surgical anal canal**
  - Measures about 4.0 cm in females and 4.4 cm in males.
  - Extends from the anal verge to the anorectal ring (Fig. 1.2A and B).

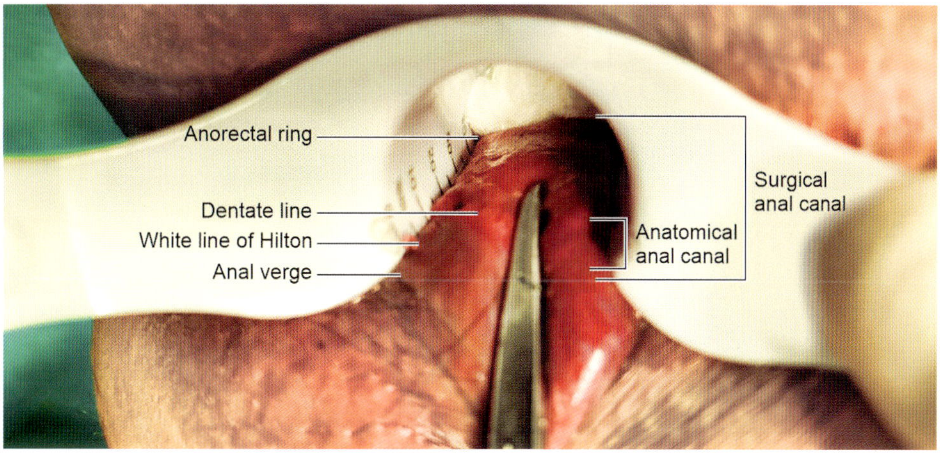

Fig. 1.2A: Proctoscopy view of the anal canal showing the surgical and anatomical anal canal. The artery forceps indicate the upper part of the anal canal

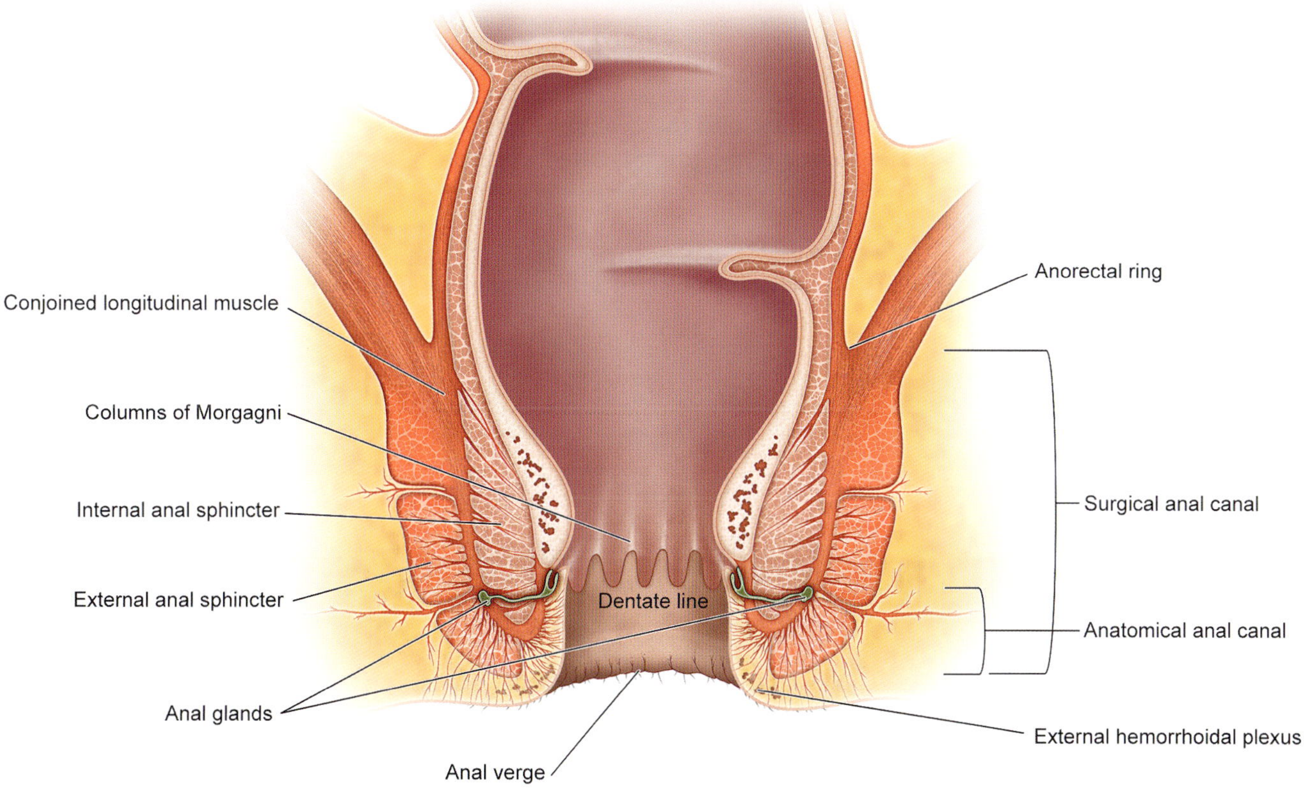

Fig. 1.2B: Diagrammatic representation of anatomical and surgical anal canal

INTERIOR OF ANAL CANAL

It is divided into three zones (Fig. 1.3A and B).

1. Upper Zone

The upper zone lies between the anorectal ring and the dentate line and is lined by columnar epithelium. It is approximately 2.5 cm long and comprises of:

- Columns of Morgagni
- Anal valves
- Anal sinus/crypts
- Pectinate/dentate line
- Anal papillae
- Anal cushions

2. Middle Zone

The middle zone lies between the dentate line and the intersphincteric groove (white line of Hilton). This is also known as the intermediate zone or area of pectin. It is lined by anoderm and is about 15 mm long.

3. Lower Cutaneous Zone

The lower cutaneous zone lies between the white line of Hilton and the perianal skin. It is approximately 8 mm long.

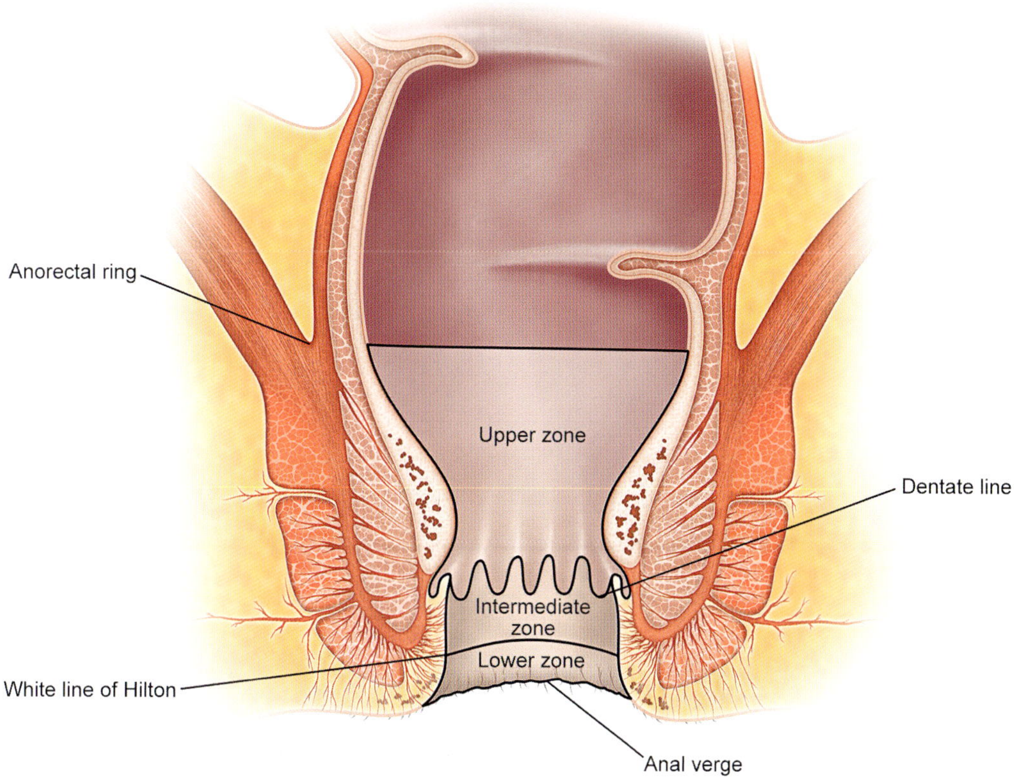

Fig. 1.3A: Three zones of the interior of the anal canal

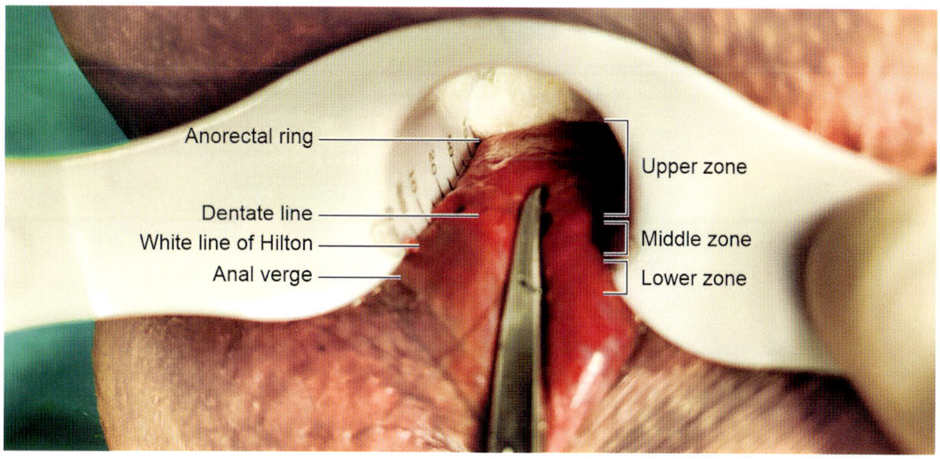

Fig. 1.3B: Proctoscopy view of the interior of the anal canal

UPPER ZONE–CONTENTS

Columns of Morgagni

- These are 12–16 vertical folds produced by the infoldings of the mucous membrane.
- These are separated by another furrow called anal sinuses.
- The mucosal membrane epithelium comprises cuboidal cells that transform into columnar cells in the rectal mucosa present above (Fig. 1.4A and B).

Surgical Significance

Below the columns of Morgagni, anal crypts are present where the ducts of anal glands open.

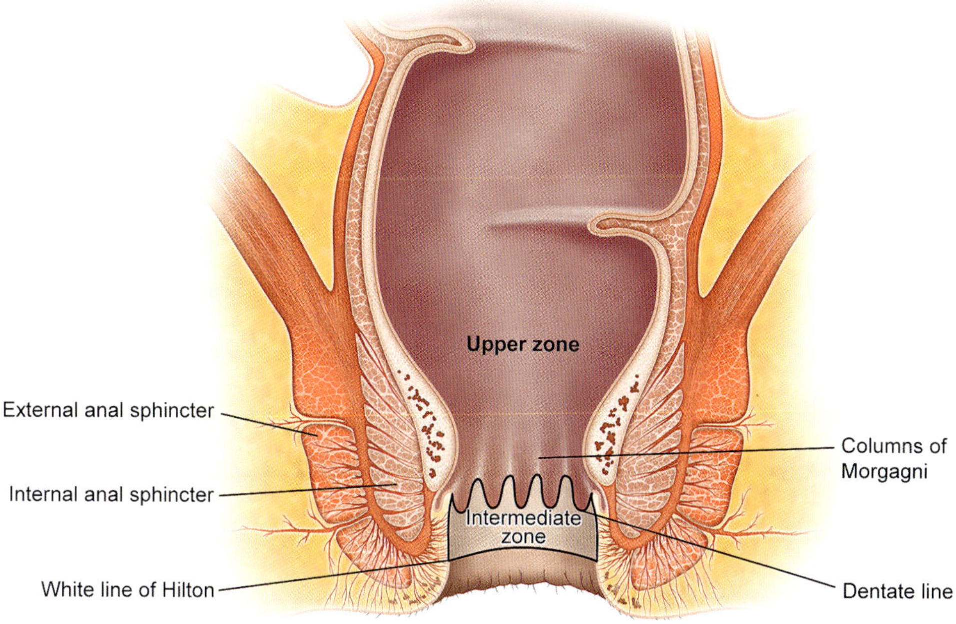

Fig. 1.4A: Diagrammatic representation of columns of Morgagni

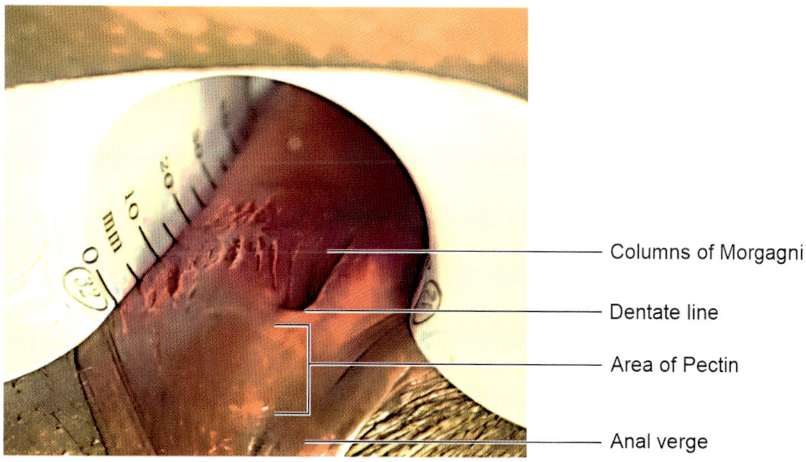

Fig. 1.4B: Proctoscopy view of columns of Morgagni

Anal Valves

- Anal valves are small transverse folds of the mucous membrane that join the lower ends of columns of Morgagni (Fig. 1.5). These valves are 2 cm cranial to the anus.
- The valves and sinuses are more prominent on the posterior wall of the anal canal (Fig. 1.5).

Surgical Significance

Chronic constipation can cause tearing of the anal valves up to the anus, leading to anal fissures.

Anal Sinuses/Crypts

- Anal crypts are small recesses between neighbouring anal columns and behind the anal valves. They vary in number, shape, and depth.
- Each anal crypt is attached to one or more anal glands (Fig. 1.6).

Surgical Significance

The ducts of the anal glands open at the crypts. Clinically, it is the site for the internal opening in anal fistulas.

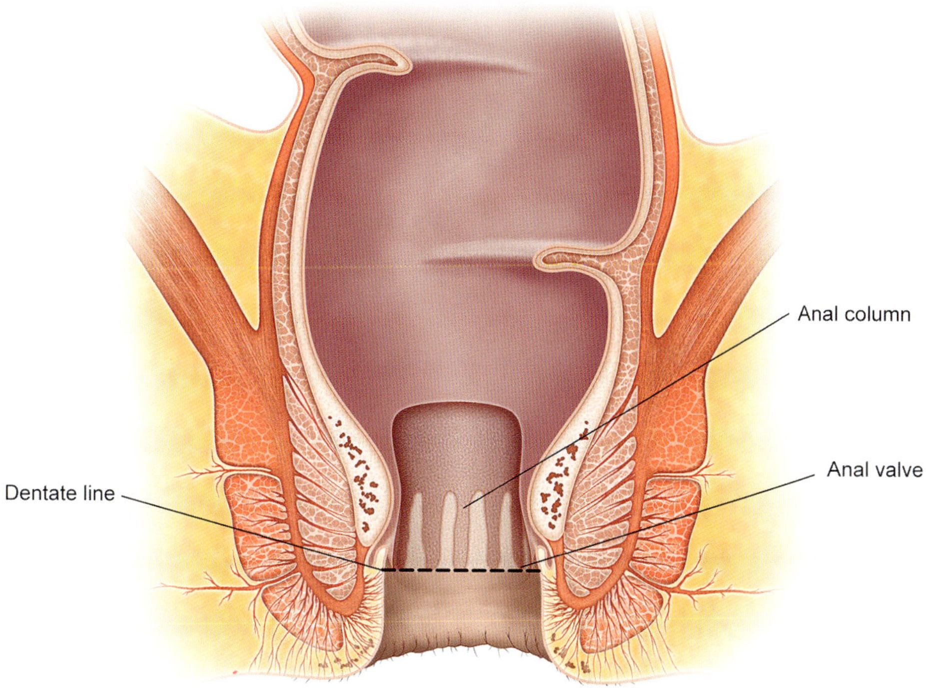

Fig. 1.5: Diagrammatic representation of the anal valve

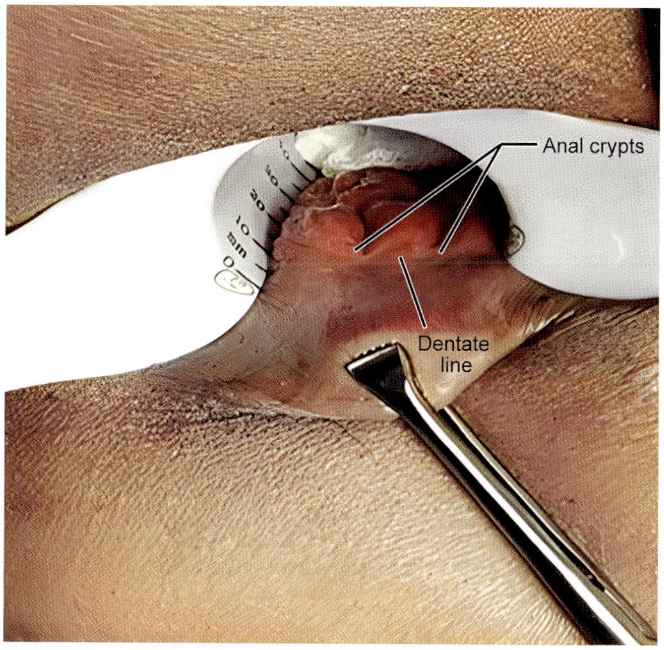

Fig. 1.6: Proctoscopy view of anal crypts

Anal Glands

- The anal glands are around 6–8 in number and are primarily located posteriorly.
- The ducts of the anal glands open at the anal valves at the dentate line (Fig. 1.7).

Surgical Significance

Obstruction of the anal glands leads to stasis with the formation of anal abscesses and fistulas.

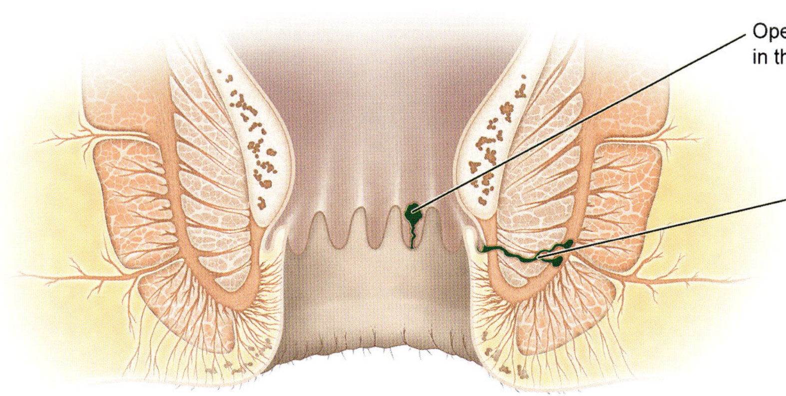

Fig. 1.7: Diagrammatic representation of anal glands

Dentate Line

- The anal valves form a saw-tooth-like transverse line called the pectinate or dentate line. It represents the junction of the proctodeum and the hindgut.
- The anoderm comprising of non-keratinized squamous epithelium is below the dentate line and extends up to the white line of Hilton. It is shiny, pink and devoid of glands and hair follicles.
- Anal papillae are present on the dentate line (Fig. 1.8A and B).

Surgical Significance

- The blood supply, lymphatic drainage and nerve supply above and below the dentate line are entirely different, which has a great surgical significance.
- As internal hemorrhoids are present above the dentate line, they are painless, while the external hemorrhoids are painful since they are present below the dentate line.
- In an anal fissure, a linear tear extending from the dentate line to the anal verge, causes severe pain during defecation.

Blood supply, lymphatic drainage and nerve supply above and below the dentate line (Table 1.1).

TABLE 1.1: BLOOD SUPPLY, LYMPHATIC DRAINAGE AND NERVE SUPPLY

	Below the dentate line	*Above the dentate line*
Arterial blood supply	Inferior rectal artery	Superior and middle rectal artery
Venous drainage	Inferior rectal vein (Systemic)	Superior rectal vein (Portal)
Lymphatic drainage	Superficial inguinal nodes	Internal iliac nodes
Nerve supply	Somatic (Pudendal nerve)	Autonomic

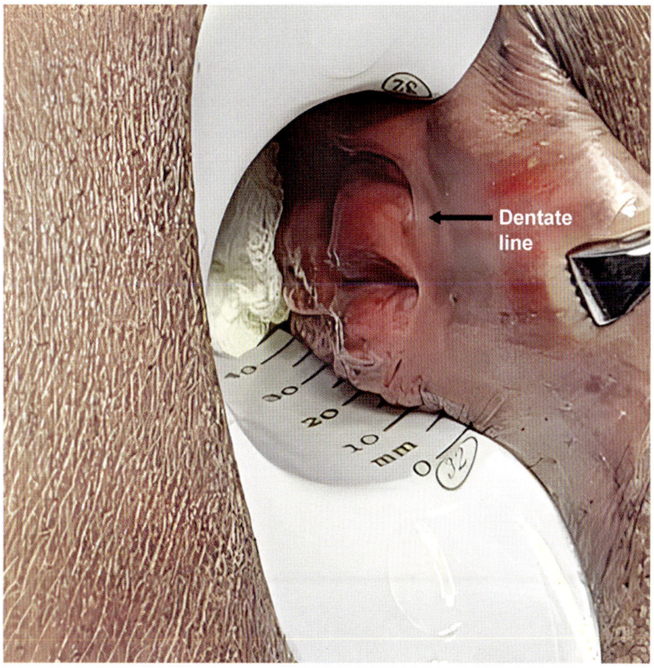

Fig. 1.8A: Proctoscopy view of the dentate line

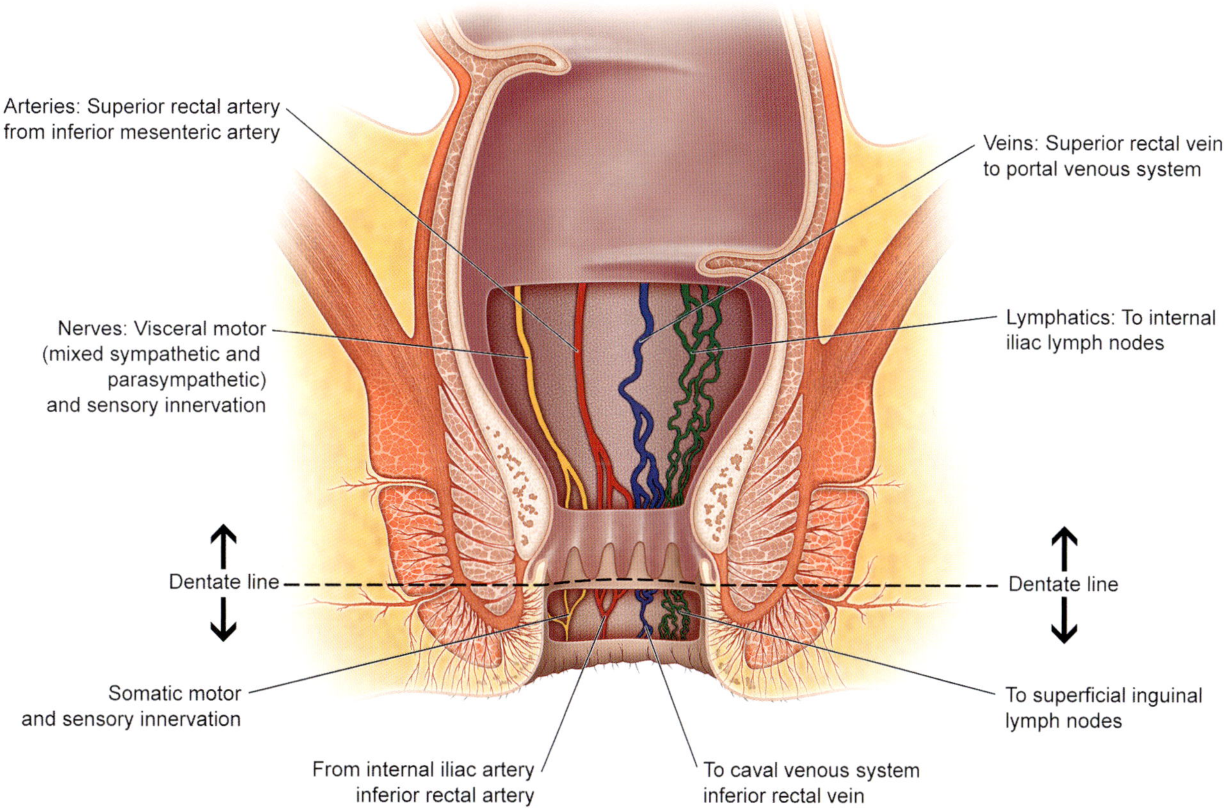

Fig. 1.8B: Diagrammatic representation showing the blood supply, venous and lymphatic drainage, and nerve supply above and below the dentate line

Anal Papillae

- They are remnants of the embryonic anal membrane. At the dentate line, these appear as tiny epithelial projections (Fig. 1.9).
- Constant irritation, damage, or infection can cause enlargement of the papillae. The condition is known as "Hypertrophic anal papillae."

Surgical Significance

Large hypertrophic anal papillae can cause difficulty in defecation. The patient has a peculiar history of "shutter-like effect" near the anal orifice at the time of defecation.

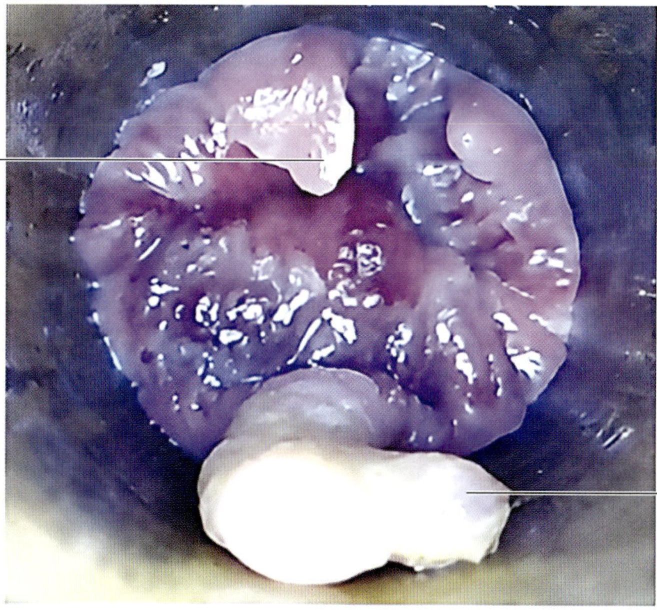

Fig. 1.9: Hypertrophic anal papillae

Anal Cushions

- The three significant cushions inside the anal canal are at the left anterior, right posterior and right anterior regions, also known as the 3, 7 and 11 o'clock positions.
- These cushions are deep purple, and hemispherical, representing the disruptions of the submucosa and extending towards the upper surgical canal. An accessory cushion is sometimes present posteriorly at 6 o'clock (Fig. 1.10A and B).

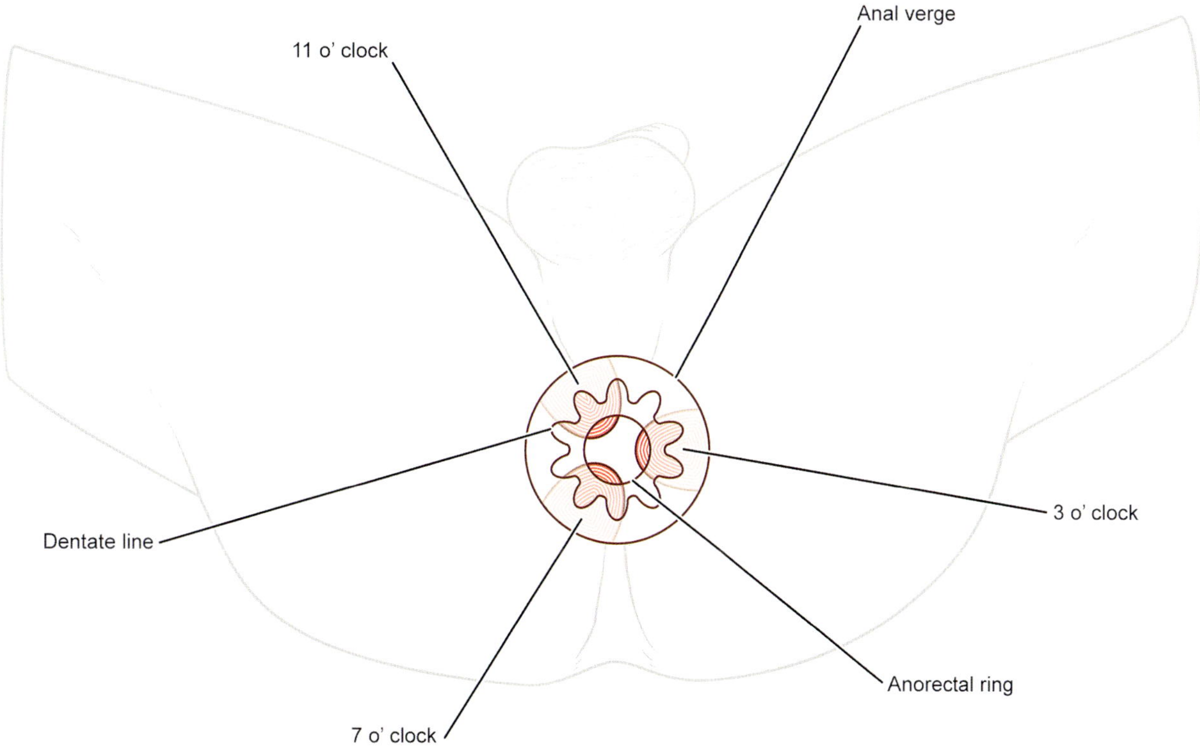

Fig. 1.10A: Diagrammatic representation of the position of anal cushions

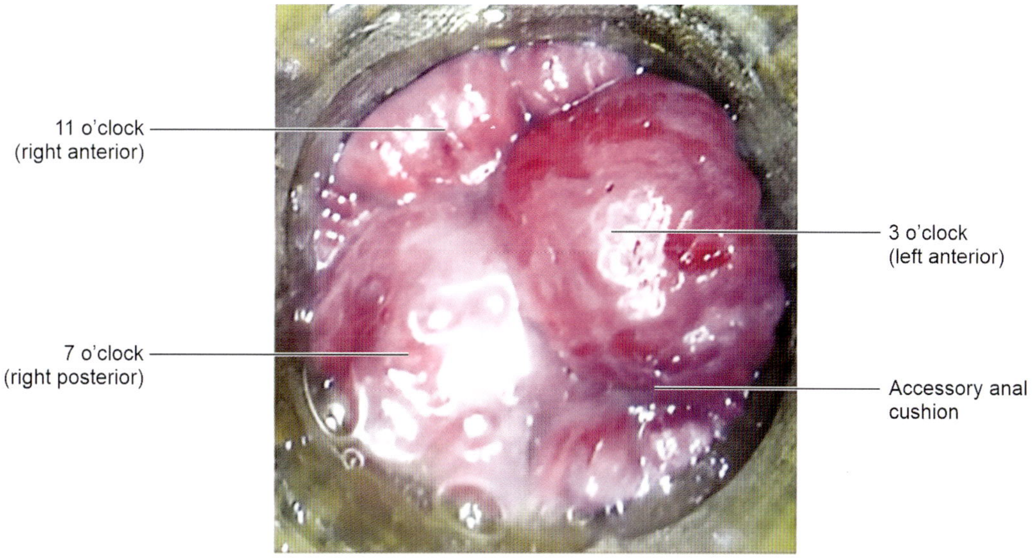

Fig. 1.10B: Proctoscopy view of the positions of primary and accessory anal cushions

Components of Anal Cushions

- *Nonvascular:* Comprises connective tissue and fibres of Treitz ligament. The weakening and disintegration of these fibres cause prolapse of the anal cushions.
- *Vascular:* Comprises the superior hemorrhoidal artery branches that form an arteriovenous network. These are the sinusoids which are lined by endothelium and form fenestrations. They form a spongy network called the corpus cavernosum recti (CCR), comparable to the penile erectile tissue. A mucosal suspensory ligament is present between the sinusoids (Fig. 1.11).

Surgical Significance

- Anal cushions facilitate anal closure to maintain continence. They maintain 15–20% of resting anal pressure.
- Inflammation of the anal cushions leads to the formation of hemorrhoids.

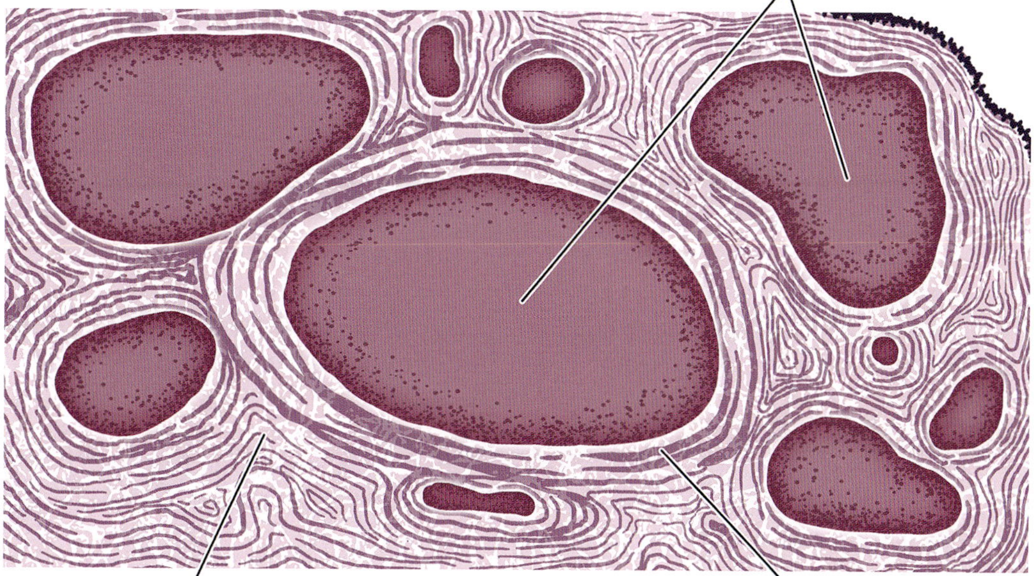

Fig. 1.11: Histological appearance of sinusoids

Ligament of Treitz

- The fibres of the ligament of Treitz originate from the conjoined longitudinal muscle (CLM), pierce the internal sphincter, and play a vital role in anchoring the anal cushions (Fig. 1.12).
- The Treitz muscle has two parts: The anal submucosal muscle, which fixes the "cushions to the internal anal sphincter", and the mucosal suspensory ligament that "fixes sinusoids to the CLM".

Surgical Significance

- The disintegration of submucosal fibres leads to the sliding of anal cushions. The hemorrhoids are classified based on the degree of descent of anal cushions (sliding anal cushion theory by Thomson).
- The weakening of the mucosal fibres leads to venous stasis, an important etiological factor for the formation of hemorrhoids (Fig. 1.12).

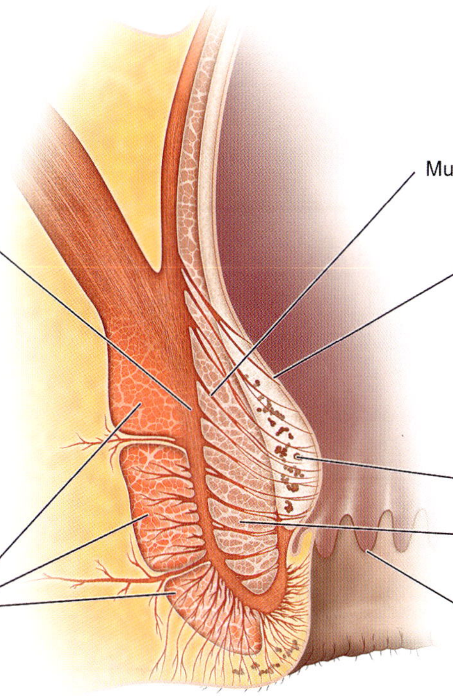

Fig. 1.12: Ligament of Treitz

Anal Transition Zone

- The anal transitional zone (ATZ) is a 0.5–1.0 cm long mucosal strip above the dentate line (Fig. 1.13). The epithelium changes to a single layer of columnar cells cephalad to this region, resulting in the distinctive pink colour of the rectal mucosa.
- The mucosa in the anal transitional zone can analyze the rectal contents and distinguish between gas, liquid, and solid feces.

Surgical Significance

The excision of the anal transitional zone can lead to an urgency to defecate.

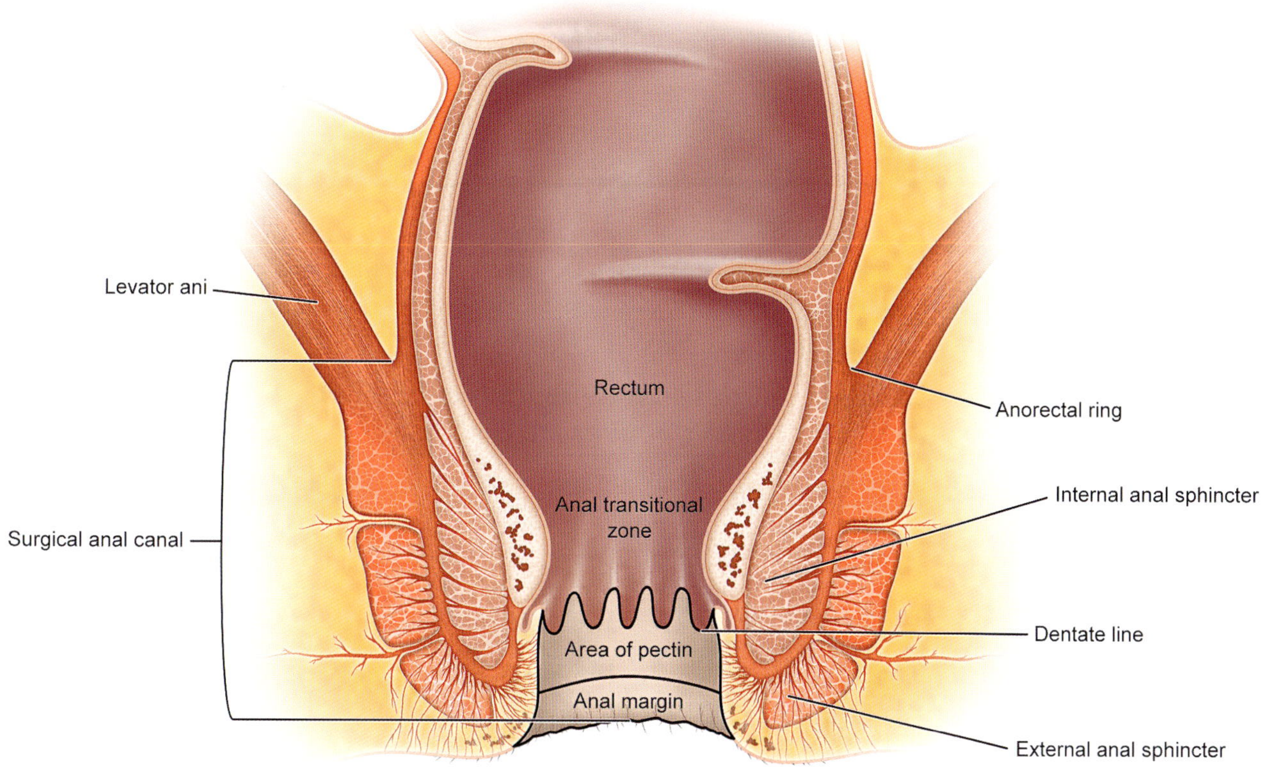

Fig. 1.13: Anal transitional zone (ATZ)

Middle or Intermediate Zone or Area of Pectin

- The intermediate zone is 1–1.5 cm long and is separated from the lower zone by the "white line of Hilton". This area is known as the "area of pectin" and is lined by stratified squamous non-keratinized epithelium (Fig. 1.14A and B).

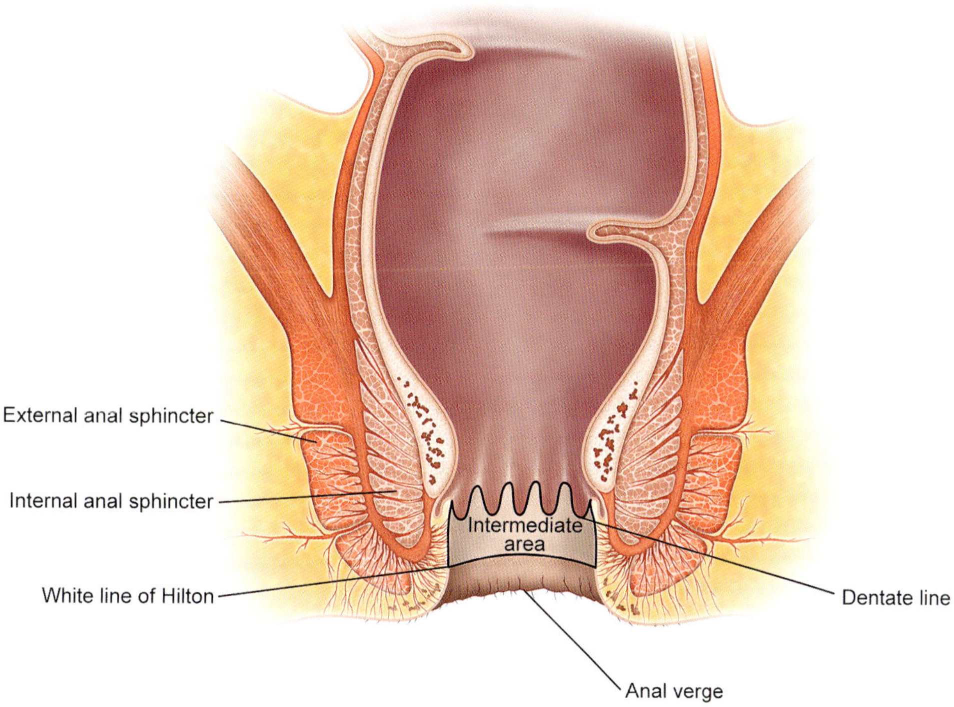

Fig. 1.14A: Intermediate zone and white line of Hilton

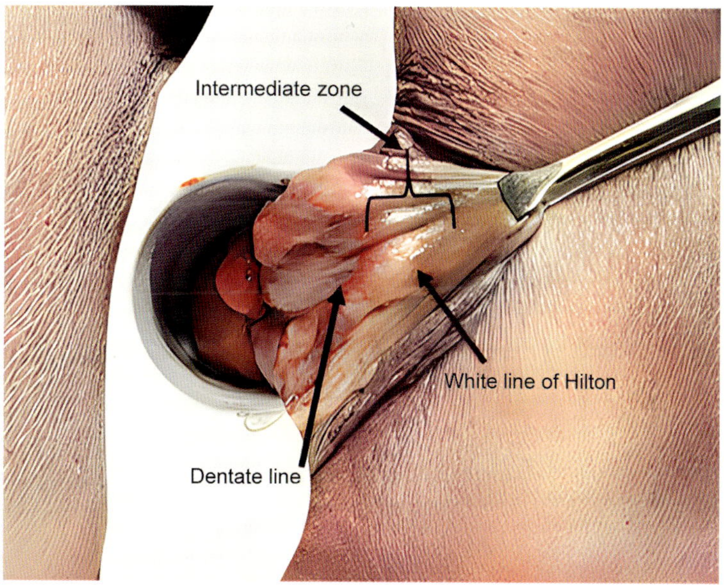

Fig. 1.14B: Proctoscopy view showing intermediate zone, dentate line and white line of Hilton

Lower Cutaneous Zone

- The lower cutaneous zone is approximately 8 mm long and extends between the white line of Hilton and the anal verge.
- It is lined by stratified squamous keratinized epithelium and has sebaceous glands, hair follicles, and sweat glands (Fig. 1.15).
- It continues with the perianal skin inferiorly.

Surgical Significance

- The internal anal sphincter in the intermediate zone is spastic. Anal fissures extend up to the dentate line for this reason.
- The "white line of Hilton" corresponds to the intersphincteric groove.
- The rupture of small tributaries of the inferior rectal vein during straining and coughing can cause clot formation in the subcutaneous tissue, a condition known as perianal hematoma.
- The lower cutaneous zone is a protective barrier between the anal canal and the external environment.

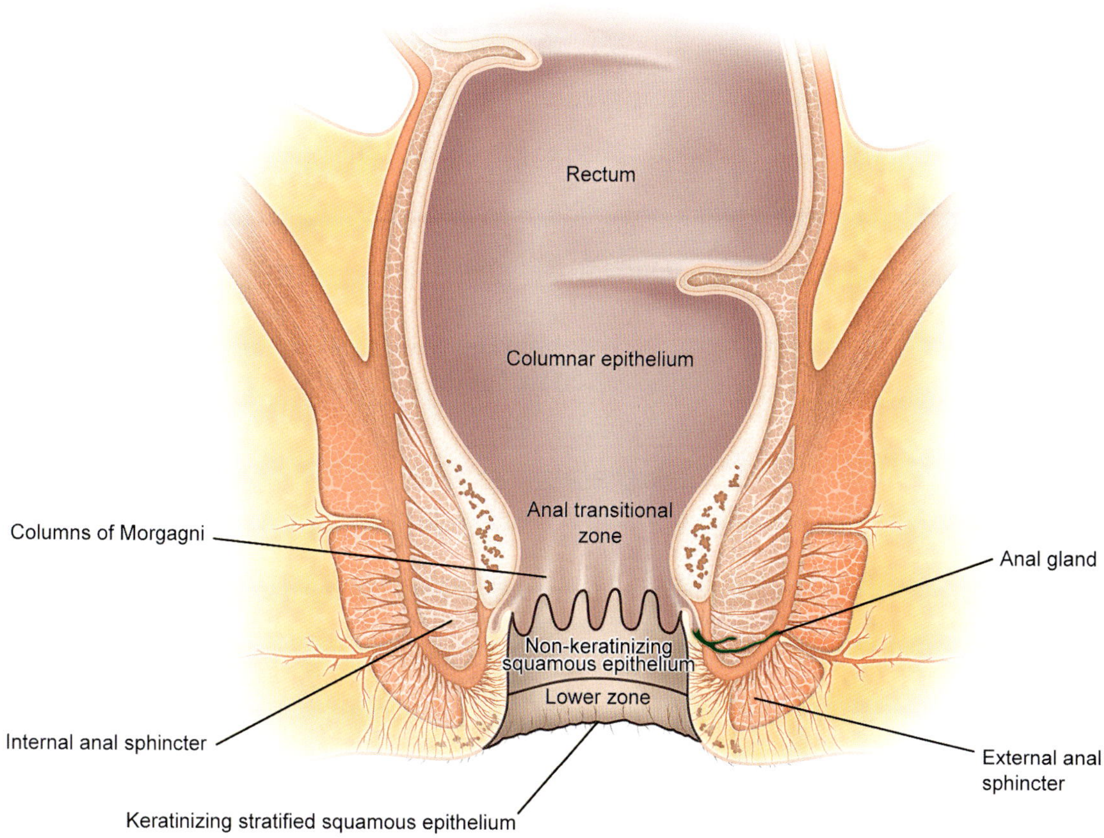

Fig. 1.15: Lower cutaneous zone

A Word about Mucocutaneous Junction

According to John Hilton, the white line of Hilton represents the mucocutaneous junction. The anoderm covering the intermediate zone is not true skin as it is shiny and pink and lacks hair follicles and sweat glands. Many authors believe the dentate line should be considered as the mucocutaneous junction (Fig. 1.16A and B).

Surgical Significance

- According to some authors, the white line of Hilton represents mucocutaneous junction. Others consider the dentate line as mucocutaneous junction.
- The junction is the landmark for fibre insertion during laser hemorrhoidoplasty.

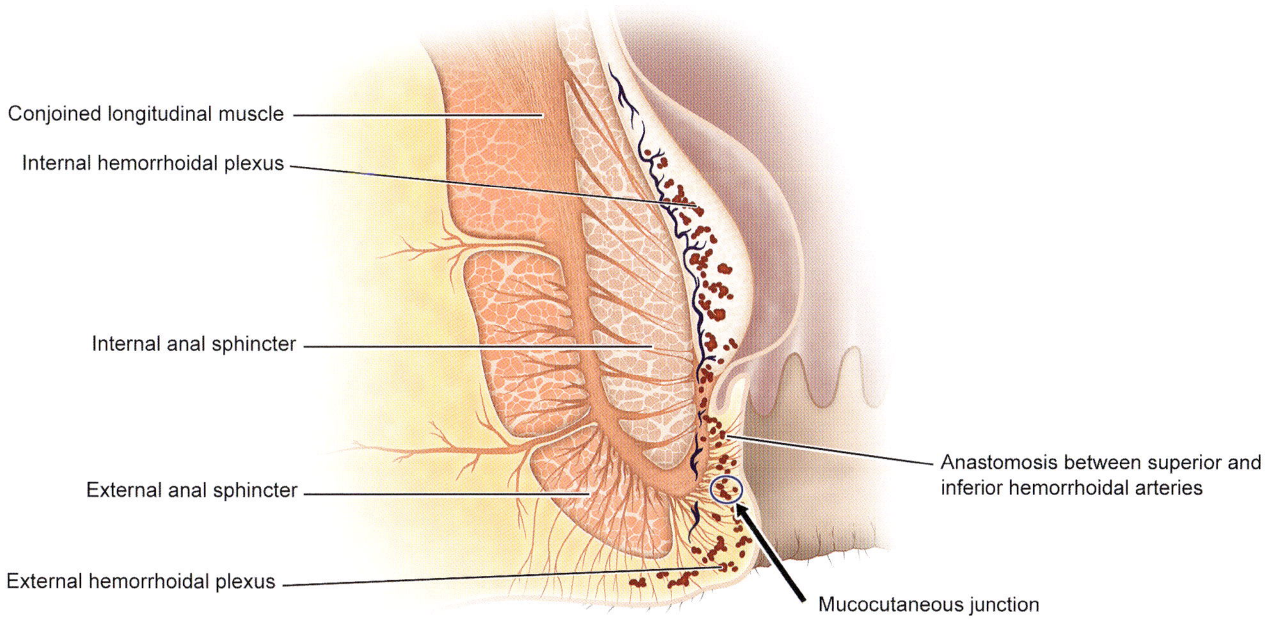

Fig. 1.16A: Mucocutaneous junction

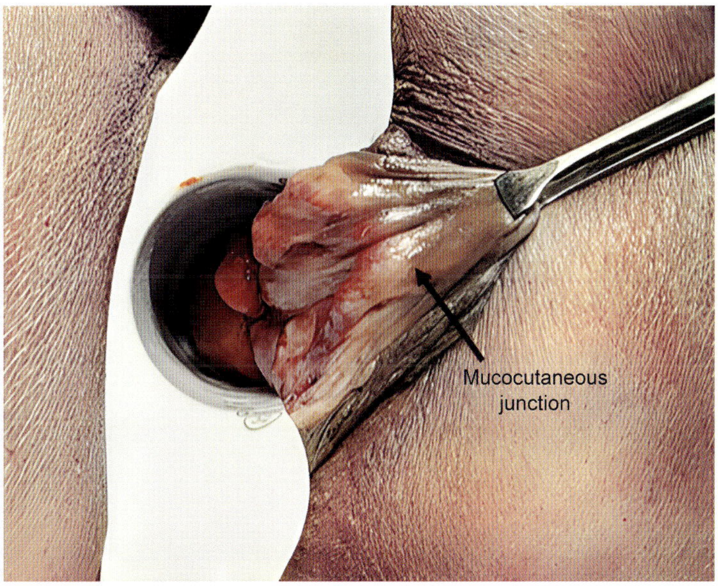

Fig. 1.16B: Proctoscopy view of mucocutaneous junction

Blood Supply of the Anal Canal

Arterial Supply

The main arteries that supply the anal canal are

- The superior hemorrhoidal artery (SHA). It is an extension of the inferior mesenteric artery.
- The middle hemorrhoidal artery (MHA). It originates from the anterior division of the internal iliac artery, inferior vesical artery, or both and is present only in 40–60% of the cases.
- The inferior hemorrhoidal artery (IHA). It originates from the internal pudendal artery, a branch of the internal iliac artery's anterior division (Figs 1.17 and 1.18).

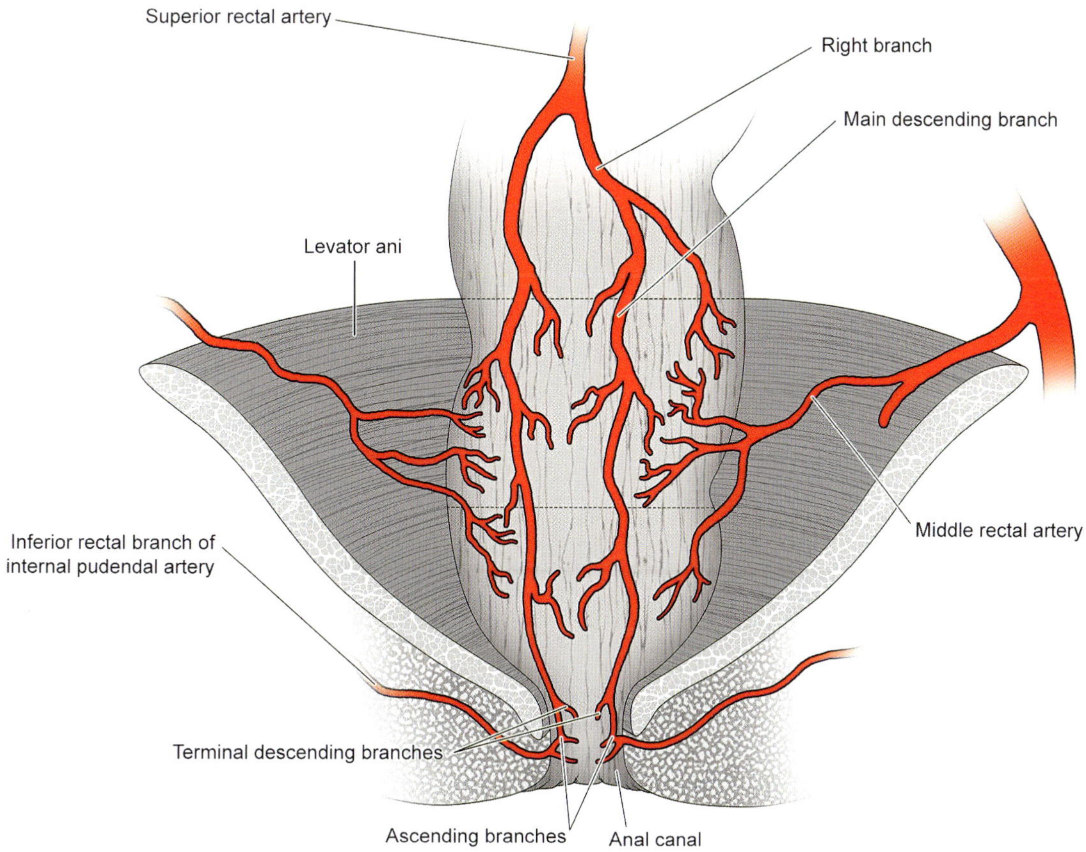

Fig. 1.17: Blood supply of the anal canal

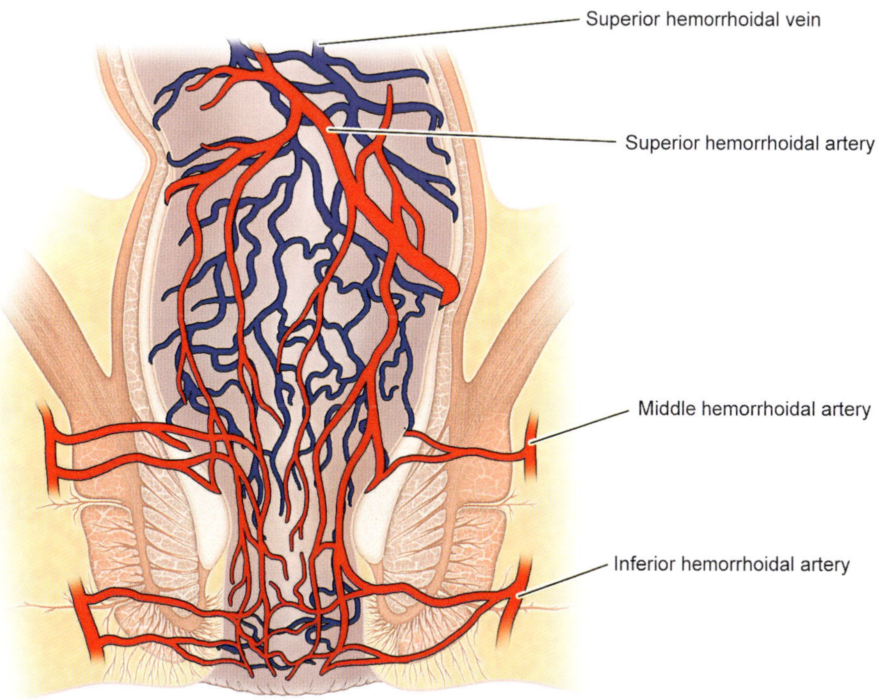

Fig. 1.18: Arterial blood supply of anal canal

Venous Supply

The veins correspond to the arterial supply. The superior hemorrhoidal vein continues as the inferior mesenteric vein to join the splenic vein. The internal iliac veins receive drainage from the inferior and middle hemorrhoidal veins. A portocaval anastomosis is formed through communication between the hemorrhoidal plexuses. However, hemorrhoidal engorgement is an uncommon occurrence. Instead, true rectal varices may develop in portal hypertension (Fig. 1.19).

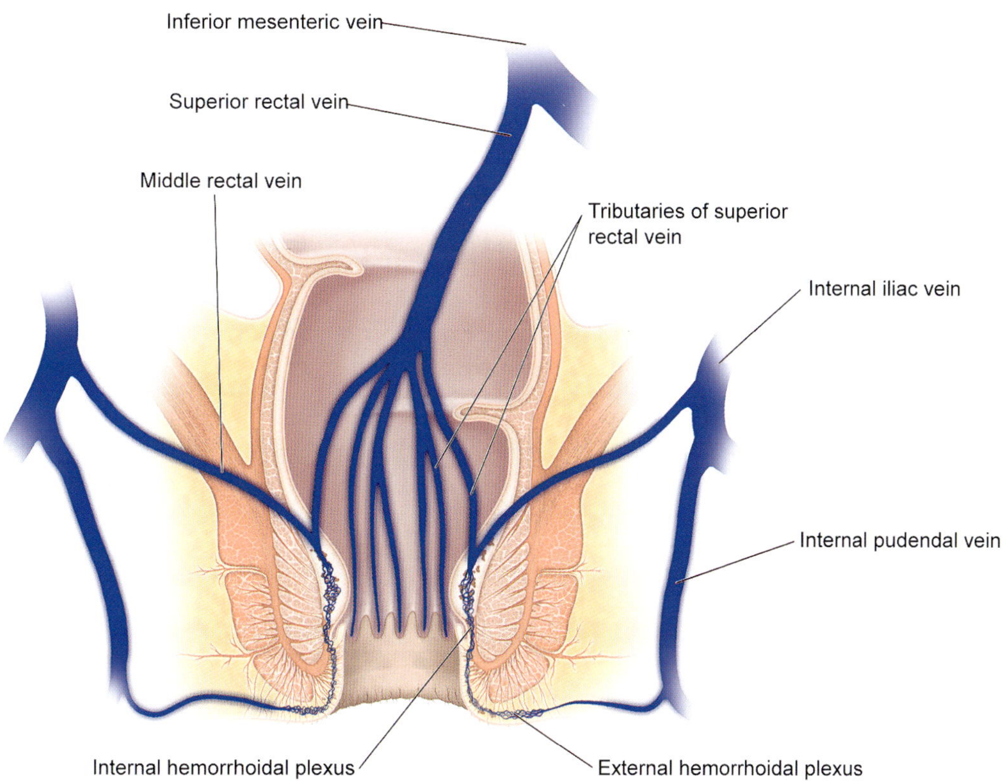

Fig. 1.19: Venous supply of anal canal

Branching Pattern of Superior and Inferior Hemorrhoidal Arteries

Superior Hemorrhoidal Artery (SHA) Branching Pattern

SHA divides into left and right branches opposite the third sacral vertebra. The right branch divides into anterior and posterior branches, which further gives three to four branches 10–12 cm above the dentate line. The left branch does not divide further (Flowchart 1.1). The superior hemorrhoidal artery branches cross the rectal wall's muscular layer above the levator ani, reach the submucosa and form the corpus cavernosum recti (CCR). A few branches of the SHA follow the extramural, transmural, and intramural course and participate in forming the CCR. The superior hemorrhoidal artery bifurcates in 82% of cases and trifurcates in 12% of cases (Figs 1.19 to 1.21).

The superior hemorrhoidal artery is the sole contributor to the corpus cavernosum recti formation (Fig. 1.21).

Flowchart 1.1: The chart representing the branching pattern of superior hemorrhoidal artery

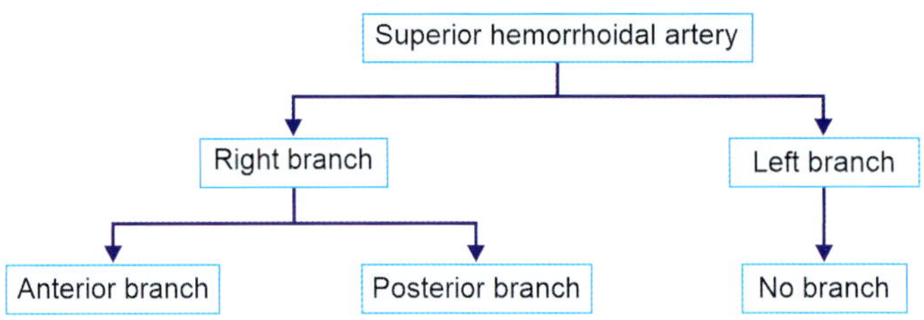

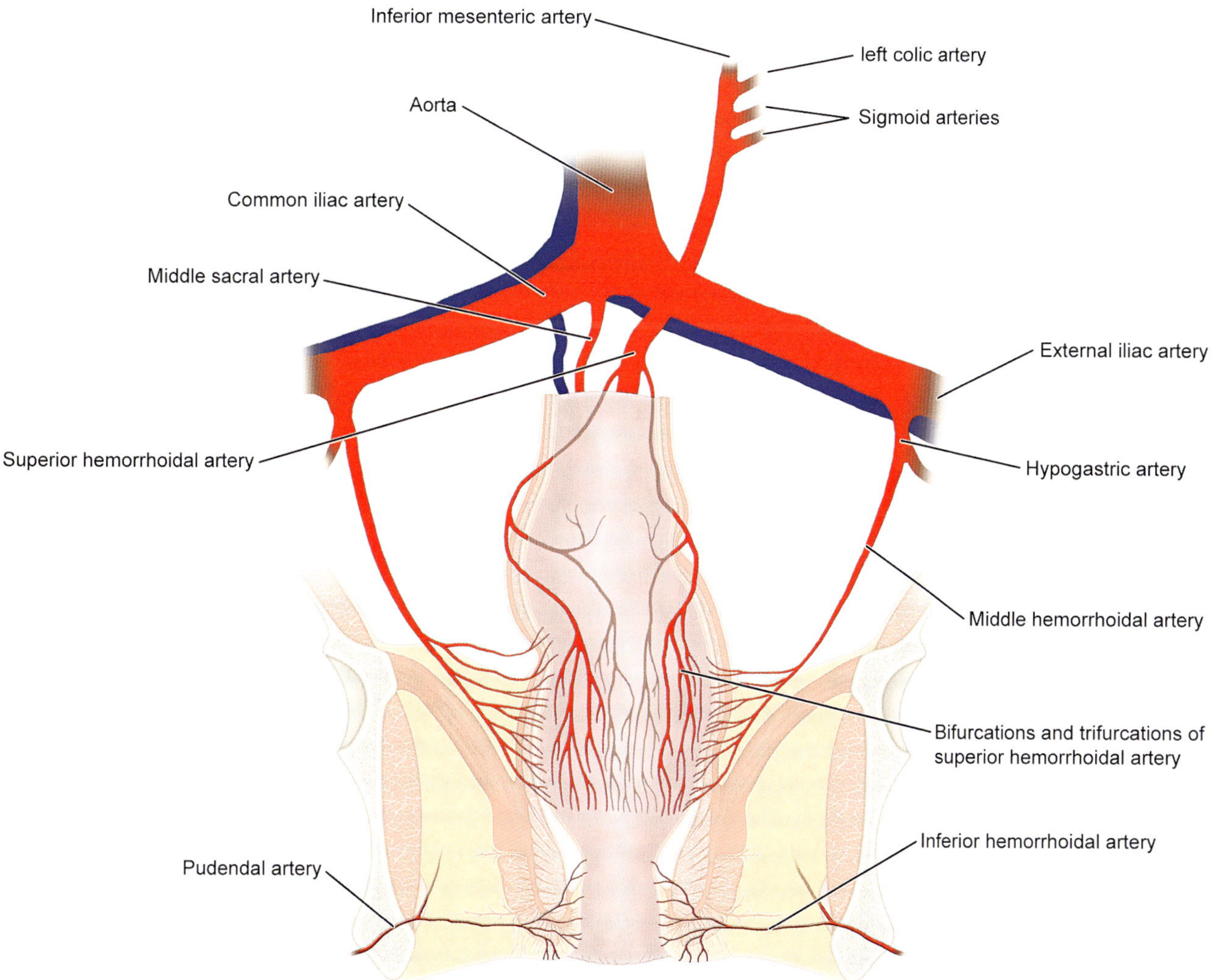

Fig. 1.20: Superior hemorrhoidal artery bifurcations and trifurcations

Surgical Significance

- The superior hemorrhoidal artery forms the corpus cavernosum recti, and its hyperplasia leads to the formation of hemorrhoids (Figs 1.21 and 1.22).
- The posterolateral branches arising from SHA are extremely high at the level of the anorectal ring. Thus, it is impossible to ligate them while performing hemorrhoidal artery ligation (Fig. 1.22).
- Two surgical procedures effectively take care of CCR in hemorrhoidal disease; one is hemorrhoidal artery ligation with laser hemorrhoidoplasty, and the other is excisional hemorrhoidectomy.

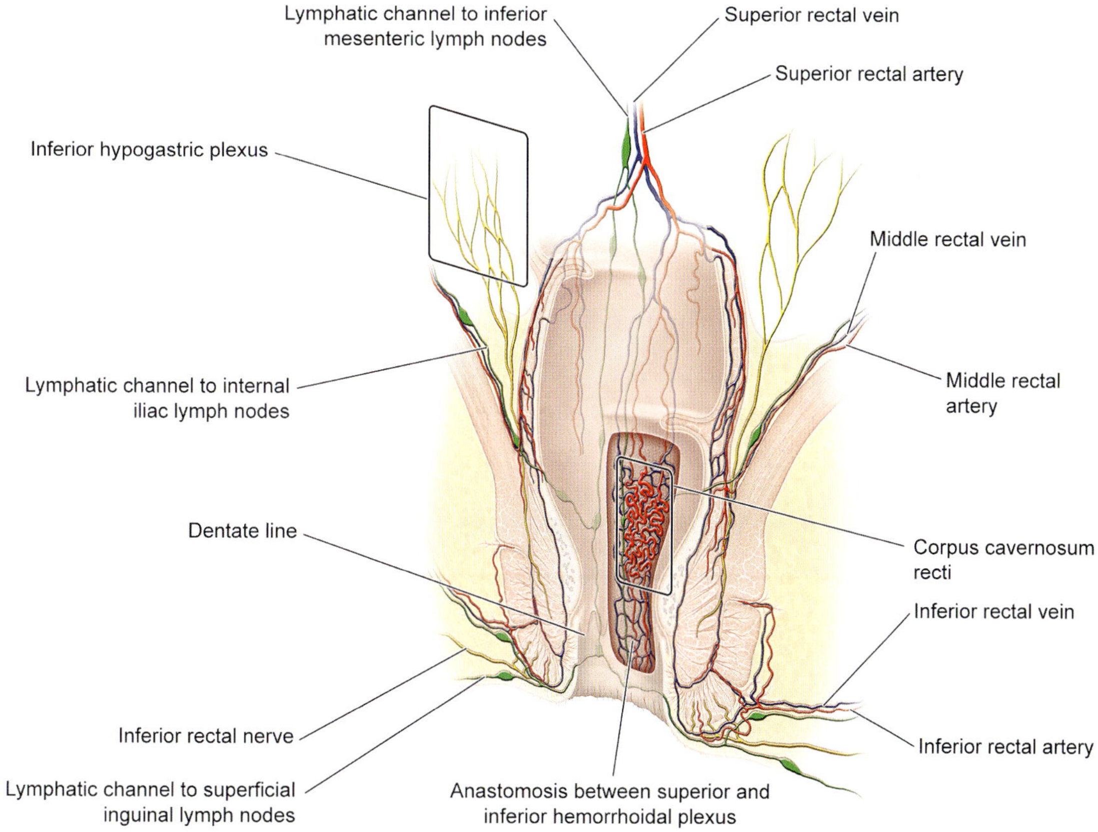

Fig. 1.21: Superior hemorrhoidal artery and formation of corpus cavenosum recti

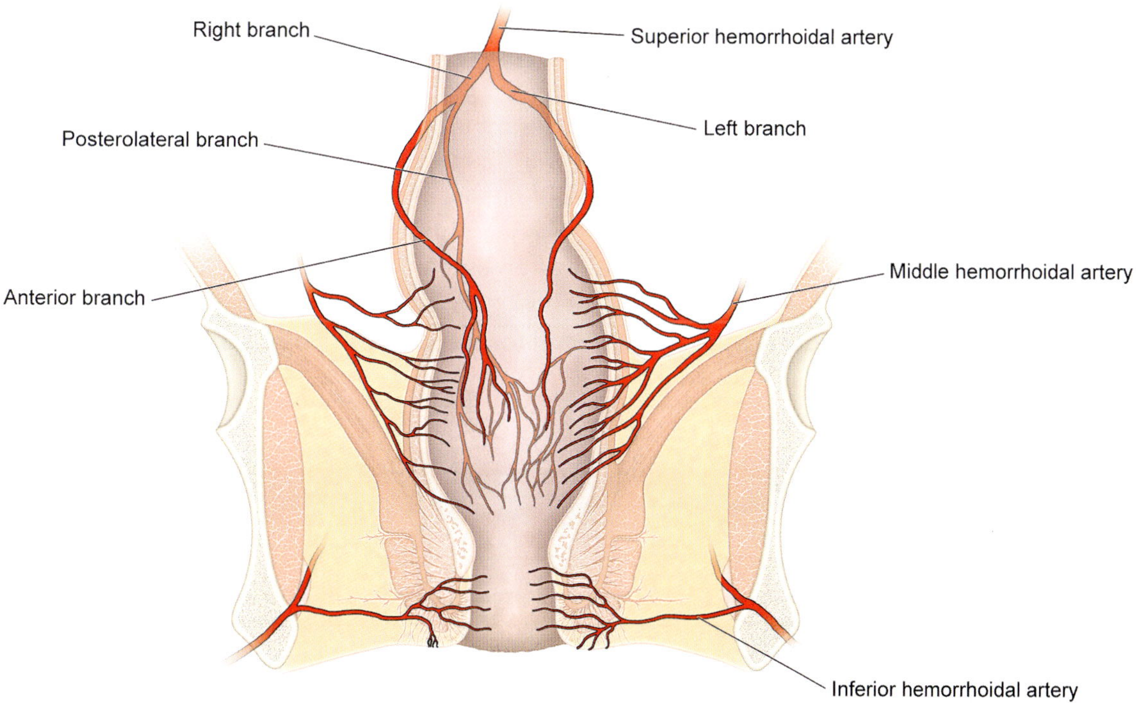

Fig. 1.22: Posterolateral branches of the superior hemorrhoidal artery

Inferior Hemorrhoidal Artery (IHA) Branching Pattern

The IHA has three main branches.

First branch: Directed posteriorly and upwards and supplies to the levator ani muscles, the adjacent portion of obturator internus and gluteus maximus.

Second branch: Directed towards the posterior aspect of anal canal musculature. It gives branches supplying the anococcygeal ligament and the posterior aspect of the anal canal musculature.

Third branch: This is the largest branch. It is directed toward the mediolateral aspect of the anal sphincters. It finally reaches the subepithelial musculature and anastomose with the superior and middle hemorrhoidal artery branches.

Surgical Significance

The inferior hemorrhoidal artery and inferior hemorrhoidal vein form an inferior hemorrhoidal plexus in the perianal space, which may lead to external hemorrhoids.

Anatomical Variations In the Presentation of the Superior Hemorrhoidal Artery

A surgeon must know the anatomical variations of the superior hemorrhoidal artery. Lack of understanding can lead to the recurrence of hemorrhoids in the surgical procedures which are based on the principle of dearterialization.

- The significance of the superior hemorrhoidal artery lies in its crucial role in maintaining the blood supply to the rectum and anal canal and its relevance in the context of hemorrhoids and related surgical procedures.
- Procedures like Doppler-guided hemorrhoidal artery ligations and transanal suture hemorrhoidopexy are based on the principle of dearterialization, which subsequently leads to fibrosis. Although the branches of SHA present in the submucosa can be ligated, the posterolateral branches of SHA are too high and deep. Hence, interruption of complete blood circulation to the hemorrhoidal mass is impossible.
- The extra rectal course of these arteries makes it difficult for the surgeon to ligate them during hemorrhoidal artery ligation procedures (Fig. 1.23A to E).

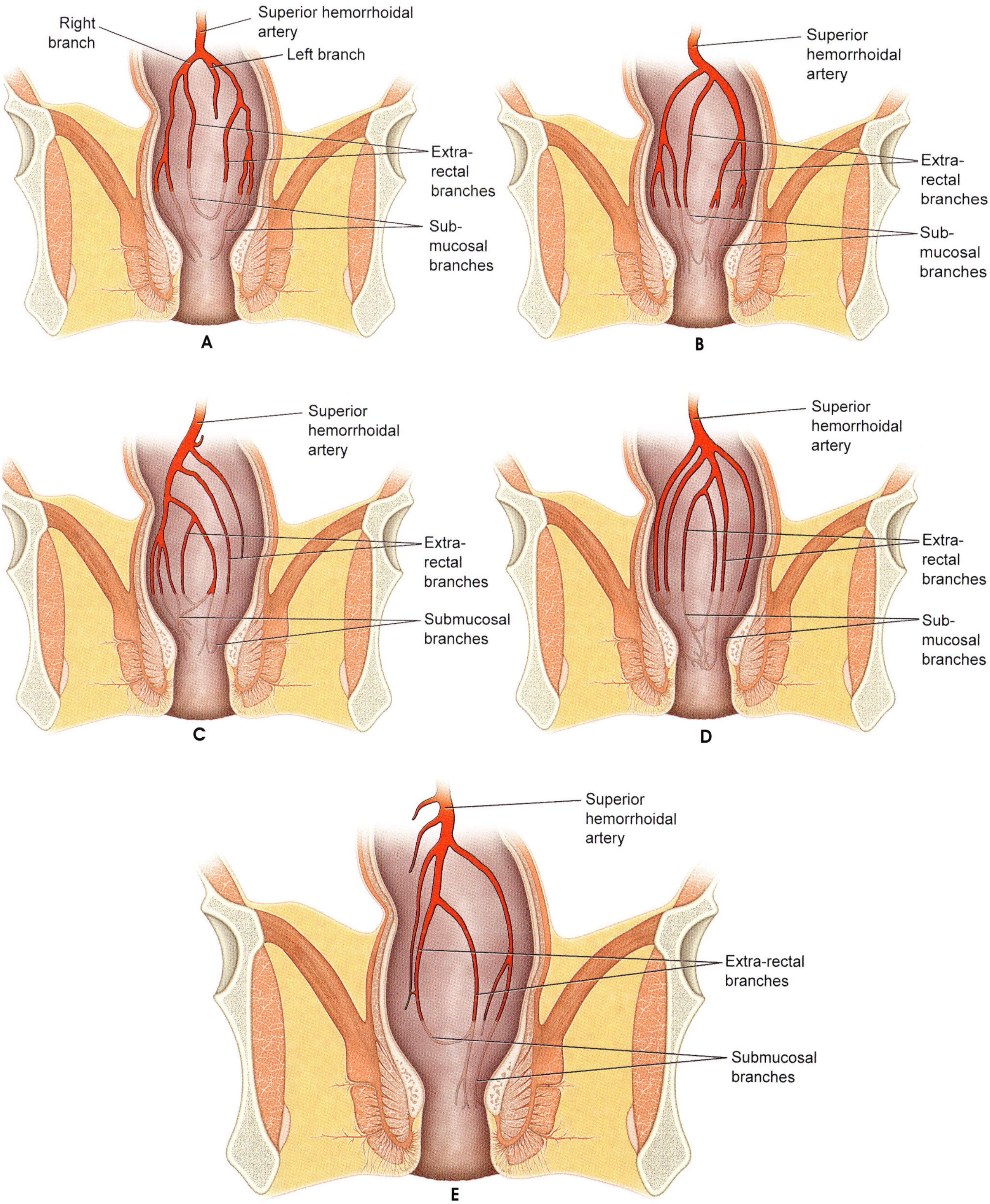

Fig. 1.23A to E: Different patterns of the superior hemorrhoidal artery and its course. *Thomson H. Piles their nature and their management*

Hemorrhoidal Plexus

Superior Hemorrhoidal Plexus

- The superior hemorrhoidal plexus is formed by the anastomosis of the superior hemorrhoidal artery and vein (arteriovenous network).
- It is located in the submucosal layer of the rectum and drains into the inferior mesenteric vein.

Inferior Hemorrhoidal Plexus

- The anastomosis of the inferior rectal artery and vein forms the inferior hemorrhoidal plexus.
- It is located in the subcutaneous tissue (perianal space) around the anal canal and drains into the internal iliac vein (Fig. 1.24).

Surgical Significance

The engorgement of superior hemorrhoidal plexus forms the internal hemorrhoids, whereas the engorgement of inferior hemorrhoidal plexus forms the external hemorrhoids.

Anastomosis between the SHA and the IHA

Although the SHA supplies above the dentate line and the IHA below the dentate line, there is an anastomosis between them below the dentate line, which can lead to internal–external hemorrhoids (Fig. 1.25).

Surgical Significance

- The anastomosis between SHA and IHA is present below the dentate line.
- It contributes to the formation of intero-external hemorrhoids. The increased pressure in the internal plexus is one of the reasons for the formation of interno-external hemorrhoids.

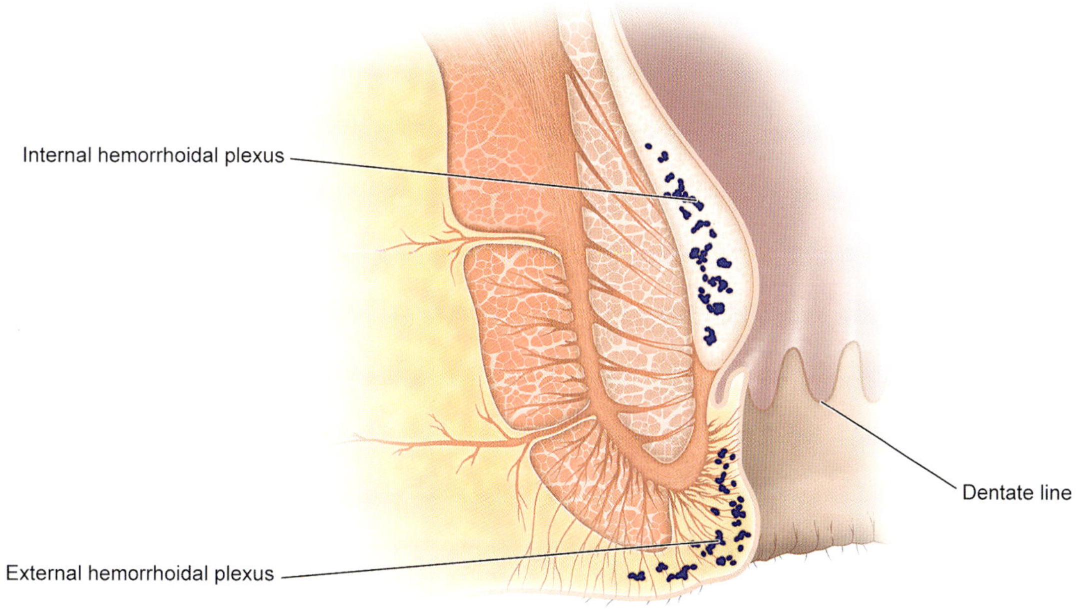

Fig. 1.24: Internal and external hemorrhoidal plexus

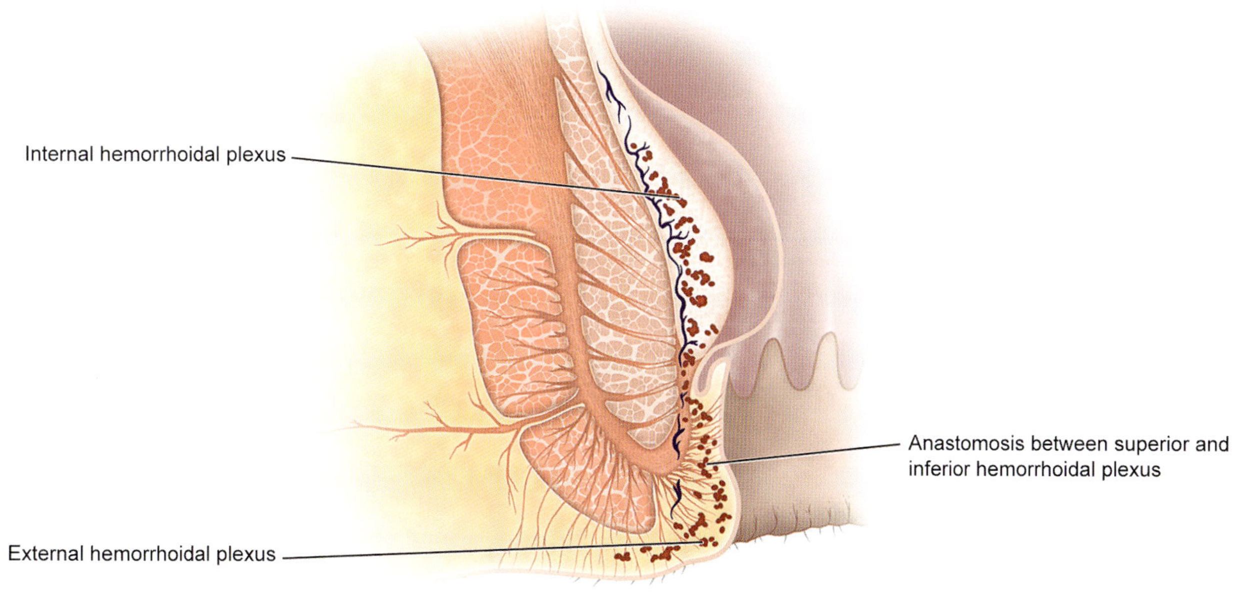

Fig. 1.25: Anastomosis between superior and inferior hemorrhoidal arteries

Correlation between Portal System and Rectal Varices

- The inferior mesenteric vein drains into the splenic vein, which joins the superior mesenteric vein to form the portal vein. The inferior and middle hemorrhoidal veins drain into the internal iliac veins, which return blood to the heart via the inferior vena cava.
- A portocaval anastomosis is formed through communication between the hemorrhoidal plexuses. However, hemorrhoidal engorgement is an uncommon occurrence. Instead, true rectal varices may develop in portal hypertension. The rectal varices are bluish longitudinal columns above the anorectal ring which extend towards the sigmoid (Figs 1.26 and 1.27).

Surgical Significance

One should always differentiate between the hemorrhoids and the rectal varices in bleeding per rectum. The rectal varices extend from the anorectal ring up to the sigmoid, and they seldom bleed. The management of these two diseases is entirely different (Fig. 1.27).

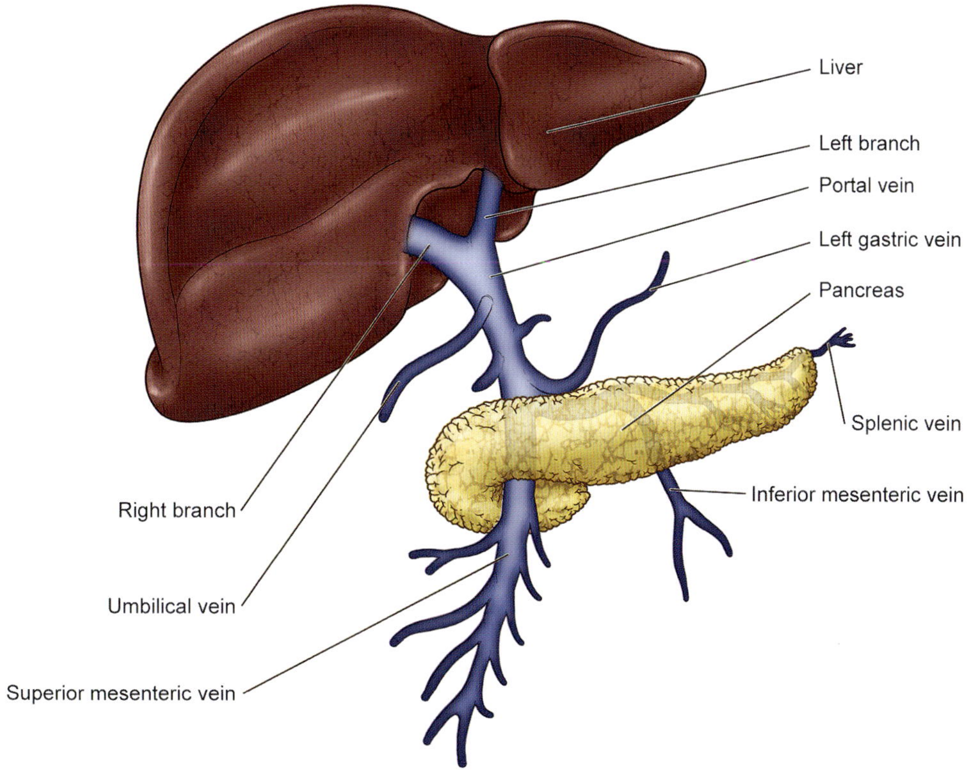

Fig. 1.26: Portal vein formation

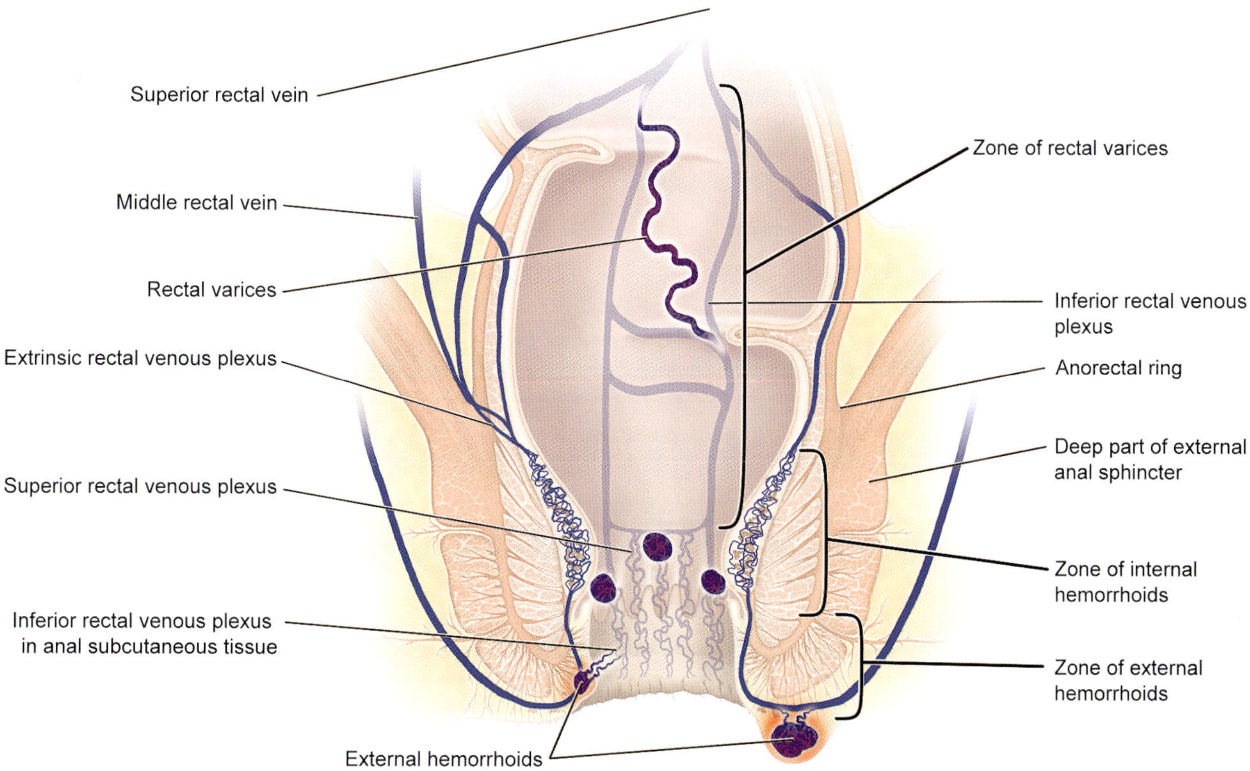

Fig. 1.27: Portal–systemic circulation in the distal part of the rectum with rectal varices

Lymphatic Drainage of Anal Canal

Above the dentate line, the lymphatics drain into the internal iliac lymph nodes and distal to the dentate line into the superficial inguinal lymph nodes (Fig. 1.28).

Surgical Significance

Since the lymphatic drainage above and below the dentate line is different, the anorectal diseases, both benign and malignant follow distinct pathways of spread.

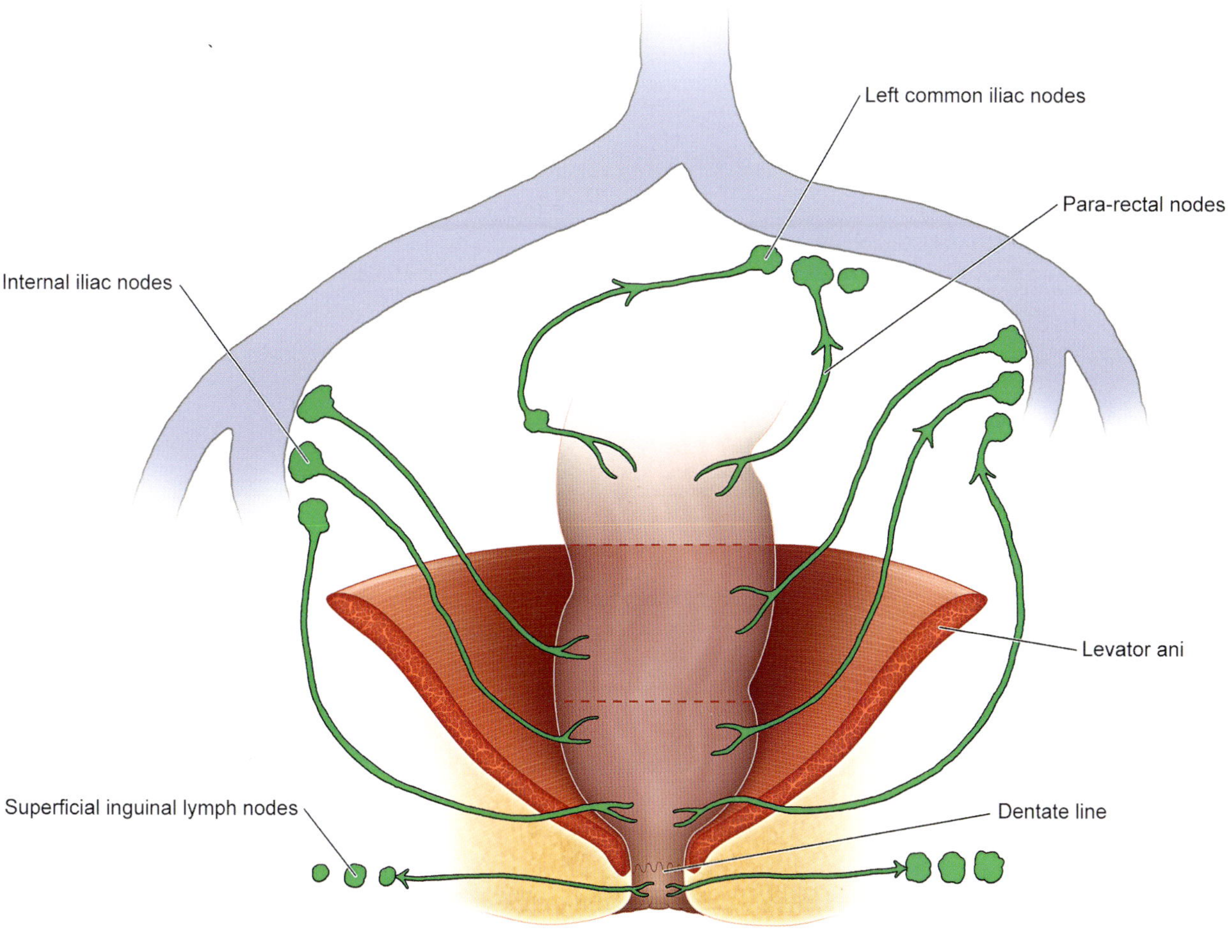

Fig. 1.28: Anal canal lymphatic drainage

Anal Canal Innervation (Fig. 1.29)

Above the Dentate Line

- Para-sympathetic (S-2, S-3, S-4)
- Sympathetic (L-5)

Below the Dentate Line

- The pudendal nerve's inferior rectal branch (S-2 and S-3)
- Perineal branch (S-4)

Surgical Significance

Since the pudendal nerve supplies the area below the dentate line, anorectal disorders like anal fissures and thrombosed external hemorrhoids are painful.

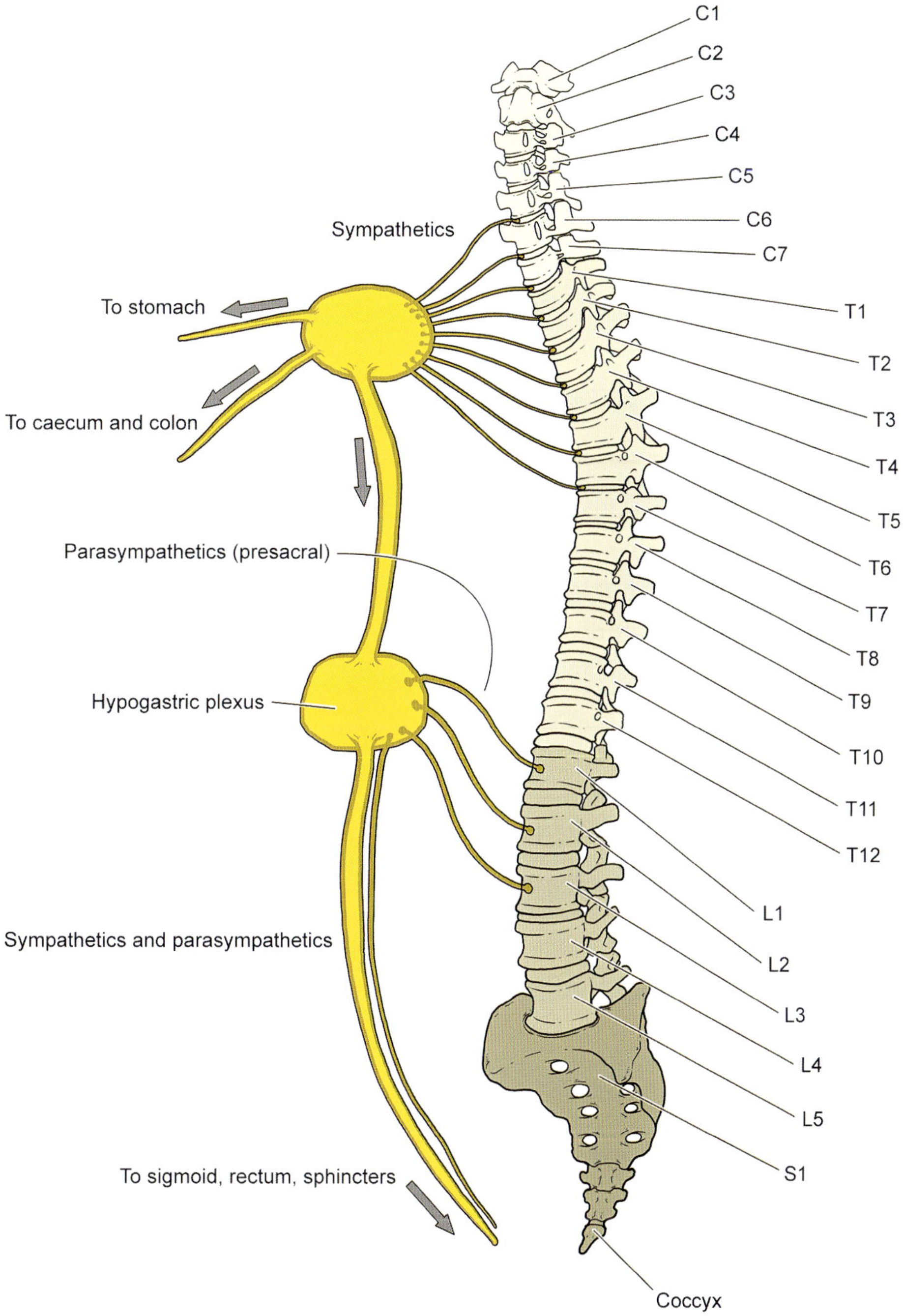

Fig. 1.29: Anal canal innervation

Anorectal Ring

The anorectal ring is formed by

- The puborectalis sling (posteriorly and laterally)
- The deep part of the external sphincter
- The fibres of the internal sphincter

It is impossible to identify these structures separately. The anorectal ring can easily be palpated by inserting a finger into the anal canal and rotating laterally like a hook at the anorectal junction (Figs 1.30 to 1.32).

Surgical Significance

- The anorectal ring plays a crucial role in maintaining continence.
- The highest part of the internal hemorrhoidal plexus lies close to the anorectal ring.
- Care must be taken to avoid injury to the anorectal ring during fistula surgeries, as it may cause fecal incontinence.

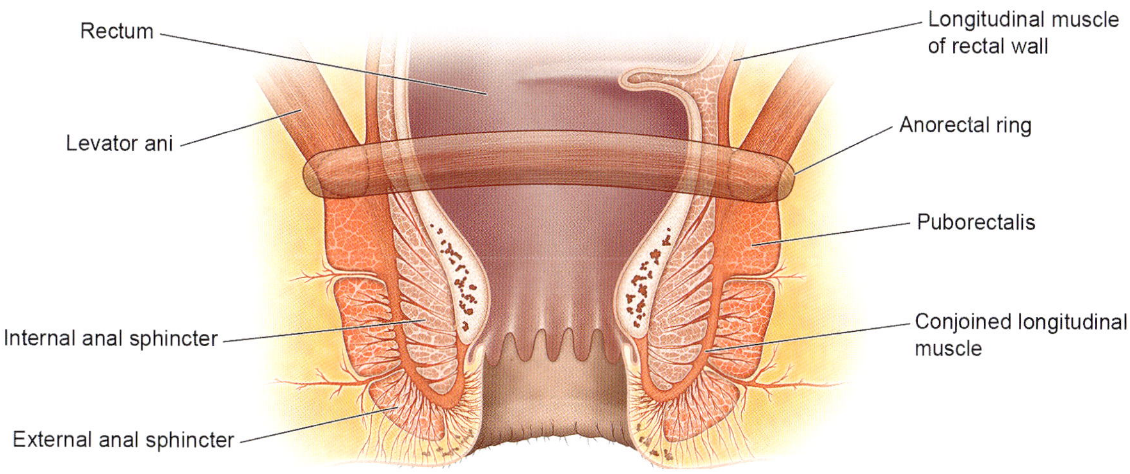

Fig. 1.30: Anorectal ring

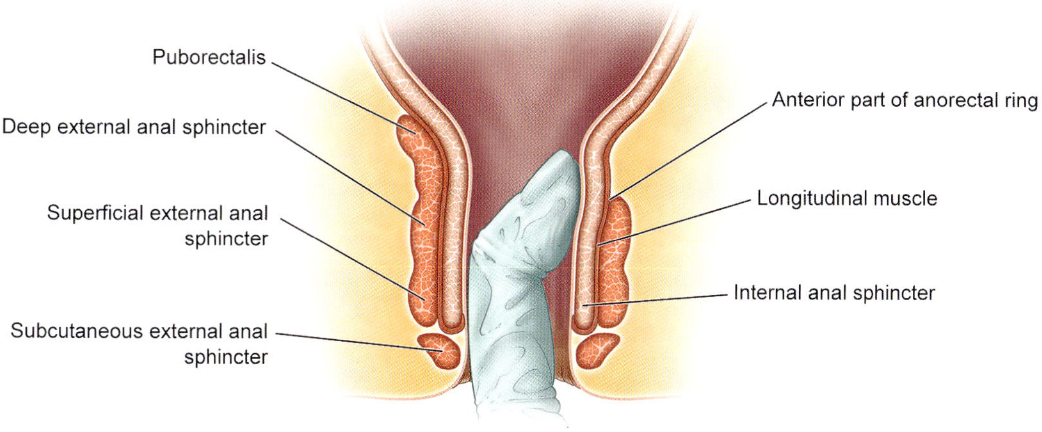

Fig. 1.31: Palpation of the anterior part of the anorectal ring

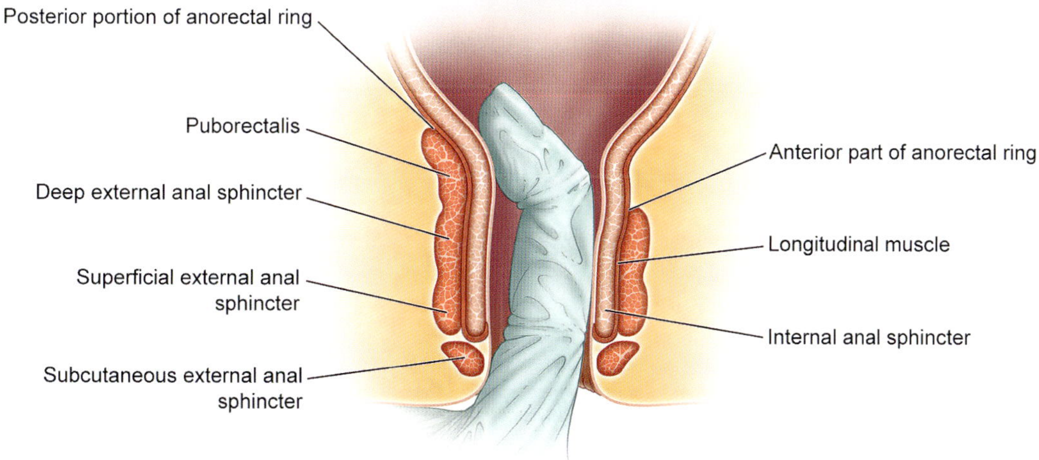

Fig. 1.32: Palpation of the posterior part of the anorectal ring

Anorectal Angle

The anorectal junction is U-shaped, formed by a puborectalis muscle sling. Usually, the anorectal angle is 90 degrees but becomes 120 degrees during defecation. The anorectal angle and the puborectalis ensure faecal continence (Fig. 1.33).

TABLE 1.2: IMPORTANT ANATOMICAL LANDMARKS DURING ANORECTAL SURGICAL PROCEDURES	
Dentate line	An important landmark while treating haemorrhoids and anal fistula. The surgical procedures below the dentate line cause severe pain due to pudendal nerve innervation.
Intersphincteric groove	Serves as a marker for anal fissure during lateral internal sphincterotomy.
Anoderm	Anoderm preservation is critical during hemorrhoidectomy since its excision can result in anal stenosis.
Anal ducts and crypts	An important landmark in fistula surgery.
Anal cushions	An important structure for the development of hemorrhoids.
White line of Hilton	Point of entry of laser fibres for laser hemorrhoidoplasty.
Anorectal ring	Helps maintain continence. Surgical division during fistulotomy leads to faecal incontinence.

Conclusion

In-depth knowledge of the anatomy of the anal canal will help a surgeon understand the structures that can be sacrificed and those that must be preserved during anorectal surgical procedures. A few precautions taken during surgery can help a surgeon prevent complications.

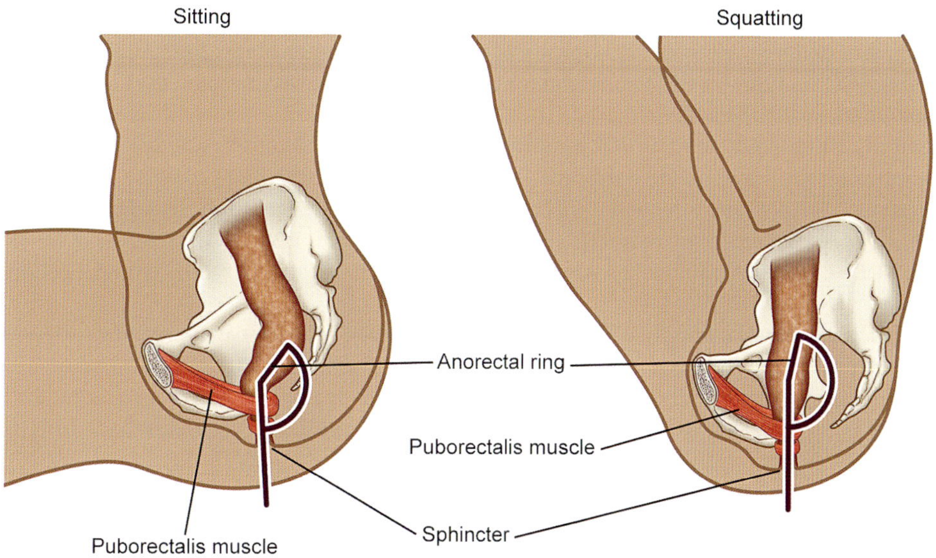

Fig. 1.33: Anorectal ring in sitting and squatting positions

Further Reading

- 1954 Jul; 47(7): 525–530.PMCID: PMC1918929 PMID: 13185975White Line of Hilton MR. Ewing.
- Ambulatory Colorectal Surgery - Page 13 - Google Books resulthttps://books.google.co.in › books Laurence R. Sands, Dana R. Sands. 2008. Medical.
- Anal Canal Anatomy Updated: June 29, 2016 Author: Vinay K Kapoor, MBBS, MS, FRCSEd, FICS, FAMS; Chief Editor: Thomas R Gest, PhD. https://emedicine.medscape.com/article/1990236-overview.
- Anal canal Author: Achudhan Karunaharamoorthy Reviewer: Dimitrios Mytilinaios MD, Ph.D. Last reviewed: December 08, 2021, https://www.kenhub.com/en/library/anatomy/the-anal-canal.
- Anatomy & Physiology of Rectum Dr Minnu DevMS | Obstetrics & Gynaecology | Dr SMCSI Medical College https://www.slideshare.net/MinnuDev/anatomyphysiology-of-rectum.
- Anatomy-anus, and rectum Carlton M. Noll and Frank D. Stanton https://www.topratedoctor.com/anal-rectal-anatomy.html. Anal Rectal Anatomy INDEX-Doctors and Clinics.
- Anatomy and Embryology of the Colon, Rectum, and Anus José Marcio Neves Jorge and Angelita Habr-Gama Page 4.
- Anus and Anal Canal Matthew R. Lindberg MD Laura W. Lamps MD https://doi.org/10.1016/B978-0-323-54803-8.50059-0.
- Goligher JC, Leacock AG, JJ B (1995). The surgical anatomy of the anal canal. BR J. Surg 43:51–61.
- Gordon PH. Anorectal anatomy and physiology. Gastroenterol Clin North Am. 2001:30(1):1–13
- G Schutte MD. & Mario Tolentino MD. A study of anal papillae. Diseases of the Colon & Rectum. 1962;5: 217–23.
- Haubrich WS. Morgagni of the foramen and columns of Morgagni. Gastroenterology. 2002 Aug; 123(2):424.
- Lee JM, Kim NK. Essential Anatomy of the Anorectum for Colorectal Surgeons Focused on the Gross Anatomy and Histologic Findings. Ann Coloproctol. 2018; 34(2):59–71.
- Lohsiriwat V. Anatomy, Physiology, and Pathophysiology of Hemorrhoids. Hemorrhoids. 2018; pp 9–17.
- Margetis N. Pathophysiology of internal hemorrhoids. Ann Gastroenterol. 2019; 32(3):264–72.
- Milligan ET, Morgan CN. Surgical anatomy of the anal canal: with special reference to anorectal fistulae. Lancet.1934; 2:1150–6.
- Seow-Choen, F., Ho, J.M.S. Histoanatomy of anal glands. Dis Colon Rectum. 1994; 37:1215–8.
- Standring, Susan (2008). Gray's Anatomy - The Anatomic Basis of Clinical Practice, 40th Edition. Section 8: Elsevier Health Sciences UK. p. 1156. ISBN 9780702047534.
- The Anal Canal - Structure - Arterial Supply – Teach Me Anatomy https://teachmeanatomy.info › abdomen › gi-tract › ana.
- Thomson H. Piles: their nature and management. Lancet. 1975 Sep 13;2(7933):494–5.
- Transrectal ultrasonography of anorectal diseases: advantages and disadvantages. Ultrasonography. 2015 Jan; 34(1): 19–31. Published online 2014 NovemberDoi: 10.14366/usg.14051. PMCID: PMC4282231 PMID: 25492891. Min Ju Kim.

CHAPTER 2

Anatomy of Anal Sphincters

Anal sphincters are essential for preserving faecal continence. The anal canal musculature includes:

- Internal anal sphincter
- Conjoined longitudinal muscle
- External anal sphincter

Internal Anal Sphincter (IAS)

The IAS is the distal 2.5–4 cm downward continuation of the inner circular muscular layer of the rectum (Fig. 2.1). It covers three-quarters of the anal canal length.

Table. 2.1 depicts salient features of the IAS.

TABLE 2.1: SALIENT FEATURES

Origin	Continuation of the circular muscle of the rectum
Termination	Ends at the white line of Hilton, approximately 1.2 cm distal to the dentate line
Type of muscle	Smooth muscle
Control	Involuntary
Divisions	None
Thickness	3 mm
Blood supply	Inferior rectal artery (branch of pudendal artery)
Innervation	Autonomic (sympathetic and parasympathetic-S4)
Functions	Maintains 55–70% of resting anal tone (anal tone helps maintain anorectal continence)

Surgical Significance

- Under anaesthesia, the IAS lies lower than the EAS as the subcutaneous part of the EAS relaxes and is displaced outwards and upwards.
- As the internal sphincter terminates above the anal verge, an intersphincteric groove is formed between the IAS and subcutaneous part of the EAS. Through this groove, the lateral internal sphincterotomy for the anal fissures is carried out.
- According to Park, IAS can be opened up to the anorectal ring in intersphincteric abscesses.

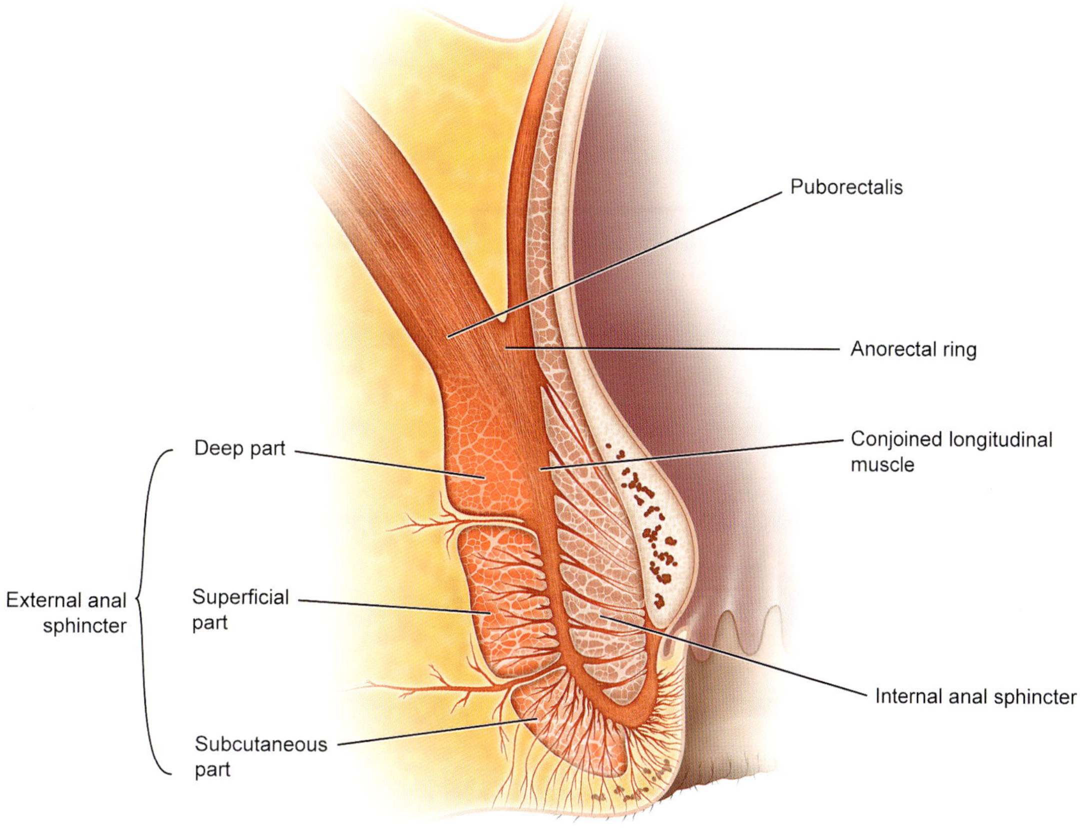

Fig. 2.1: IAS, CLM, EAS and anorectal ring

Conjoined Longitudinal Muscle (CLM)

Conjoined longitudinal muscle is the continuation of the longitudinal muscular coat of the rectum. Anteriorly, it represents the recto-urethralis muscle. The longitudinal muscle fibres are strongly attached to the (Table 2.2):

- Triangular ligament
- The urethra
- The end of the prostate

Three fibromuscular expansions surround the perianal and outer space (Fig. 2.2).

1. The inward extension is the intermuscular septum, which extends from the IAS above and the subcutaneous part of the EAS below.
2. The outward extension is the Milligan's septum that divides the ischiorectal fossa into an ischiorectal space above and a perianal space below.
3. The downward extension is in the perianal skin, forming corrugator cutis ani. The external hemorrhoidal plexus is present here.

TABLE 2.2: SALIENT FEATURES OF THE CONJOINED LONGITUDINAL MUSCLE	
Origin	Continuation of the longitudinal muscle of the rectum
Insertion	Perianal skin
Type of muscle	Smooth muscle
Control	Involuntary
Divisions	• Intermuscular septum • Milligan septum • Corrugated cutis ani
Thickness	2.5 mm
Blood supply	Inferior rectal artery (branch of pudendal artery)
Innervation	Autonomic (sympathetic and parasympathetic)
Functions	• Helps in anchoring anal cushions (Treitz ligament) • Helps in continence (rectourethralis muscle is connected to CLM)

Surgical Significance

Ligament of Treitz's muscle

- Muscle weakening leads to prolapse of the anal cushion (sliding anal cushion theory by Thomson in 1976).

Intermuscular Septum

- Prevents infection from extending from the perianal space into the cephalad submucous space.

Corrugator cutis ani

- The commonest site for perianal abscess and thrombosed hemorrhoids. Due to the presence of septa, the swellings formed in this area are very painful.

Milligan septum

- Prevents the infection in the perianal space from spreading upwards into the ischiorectal fossa.

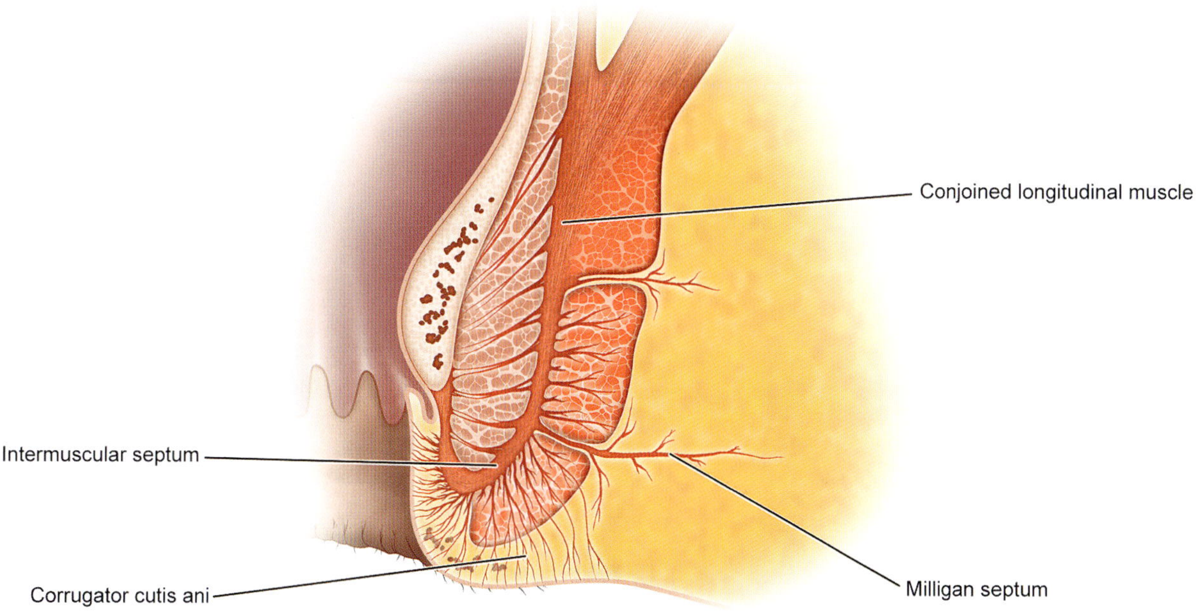

Fig. 2.2: Fibromuscular expansions of the conjoined longitudinal muscle

External Anal Sphincter (EAS)

EAS is a striated muscle surrounding the anus and the anal canal (Figs 2.1 and 2.3).

It has three parts:

- Subcutaneous
- Superficial
- Deep

Relations of External Anal Sphincter with Perineum

Subcutaneous Part

- Lies below the IAS

Superficial Part

- *Anteriorly:* Perineal body
- *Posteriorly:* Coccyx and anococcygeal ligament

Deep Part

- *Anteriorly:* Superficial transverse perineal muscle
- *Posteriorly:* Anococcygeal raphe

The deep part blends with the puborectalis muscle. This also represents Shafik's triple-loop system (Table 2.3 and Fig. 2.3).

Surgical Significance

Under anesthesia, the length of the anal canal is shortened by 1 cm as the EAS is displaced outwards and upwards.

TABLE 2.3: SALIENT FEATURES OF THE EXTERNAL ANAL SPHINCTER	
Origin	Skin and fascia which surround the anal canal
Insertion	Posteriorly into the anococcygeal ligament Anteriorly into the perineal body
Type of muscle	Skeletal muscle
Control	Voluntary
Divisions	• Subcutaneous • Superficial • Deep
Thickness	6 mm (Fig. 2.4)
Blood Supply	Inferior rectal artery (a pudendal artery branch)
Innervation	Pudendal nerve's inferior rectal branches (S2–S4)
Functions	• Voluntary control of defecation • Helps to support the pelvis along with the perineal muscles • Maintains 15–20% of resting anal tone

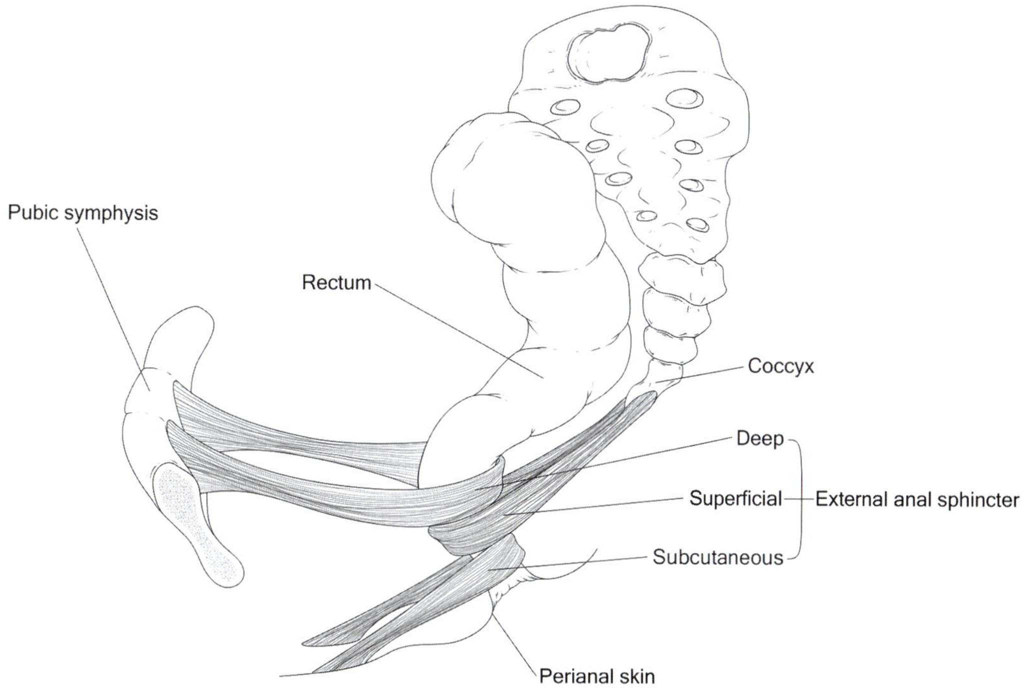

Fig. 2.3: Insertion of fibres of EAS and triple loop system

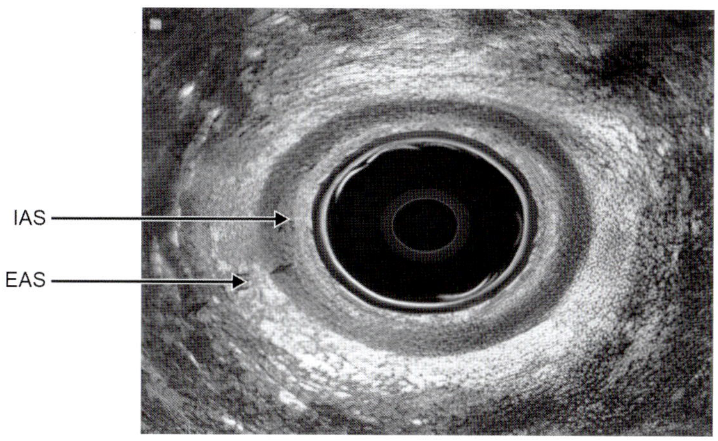

Fig. 2.4: Ultrasonography appearance of internal and external anal sphincter

Surgical Significance

In the following conditions, the sphincters can be cut without fear of incontinence:

Intersphincteric fistula

- IAS's lower part and EAS's subcutaneous part (Fig. 2.5)

Low Trans-sphincteric fistula

- The lower end of the IAS and up to 30% of the superficial part of EAS (Fig. 2.6).

High Trans-sphincteric fistula

- Up to 50% of the EAS (Fig. 2.7). Primary sphincter repair should be done to prevent anal incontinence.

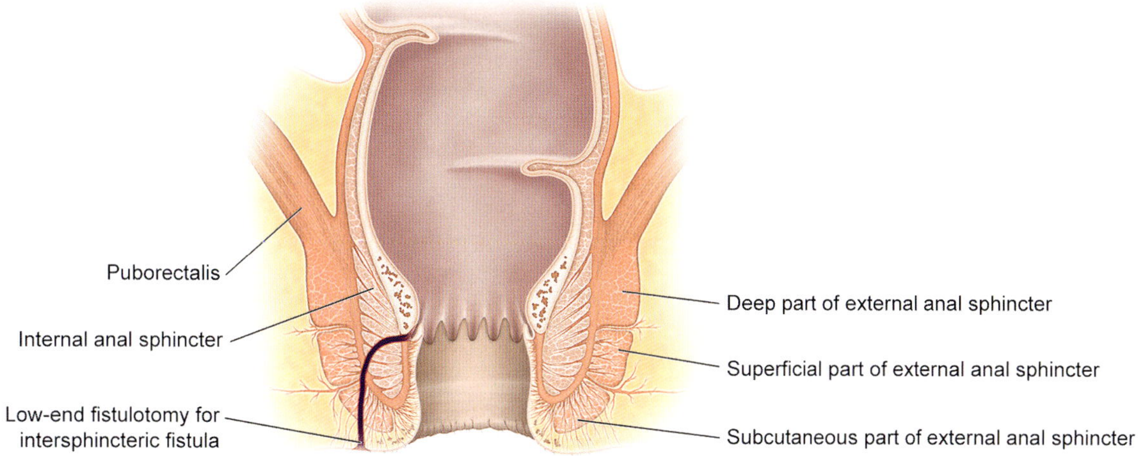

Fig. 2.5: How much sphincter to cut (Intersphincteric fistula)

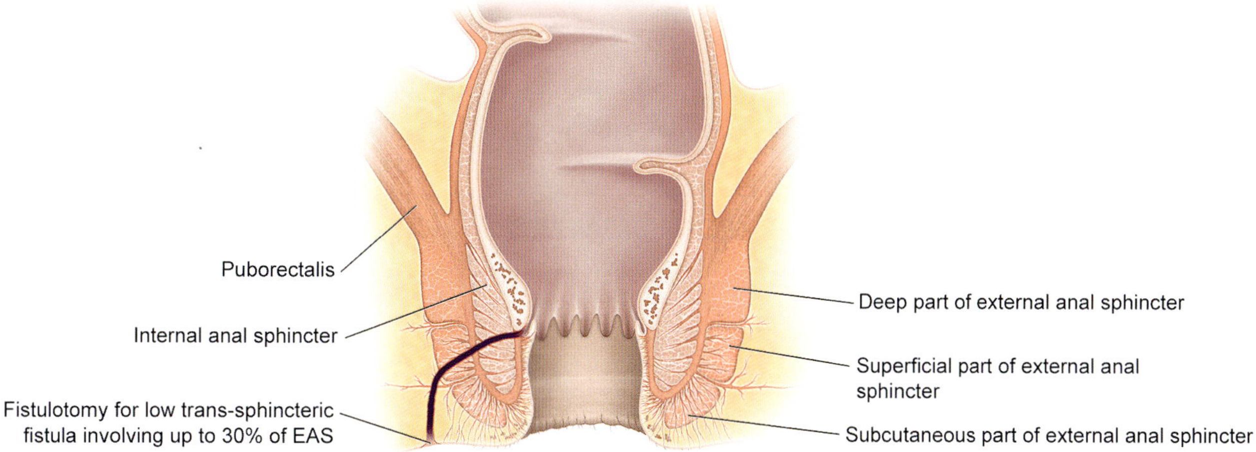

Fig. 2.6: Fistulotomy for low trans-sphincteric fistula

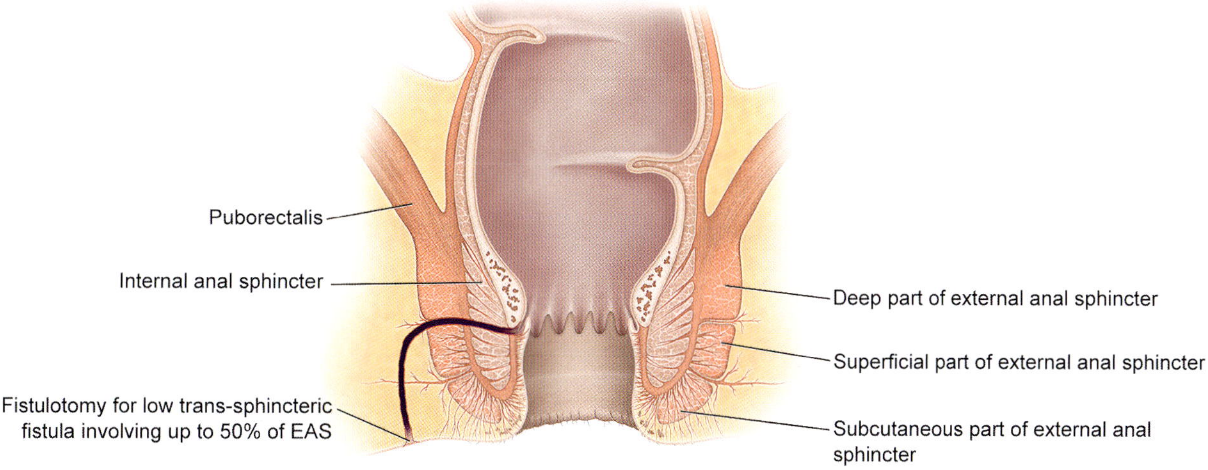

Fig. 2.7: Fistulotomy for high trans-sphincteric fistula

Intersphincteric Groove

- The groove lies between the IAS and EAS and correlates to the white line of Hilton (Fig. 2.8).

Surgical Significance

The lateral internal sphincterotomy for anal fissures is always carried out through the intersphincteric groove. The groove can be palpated with the index finger and the thumb as shown in (Fig. 2.8).

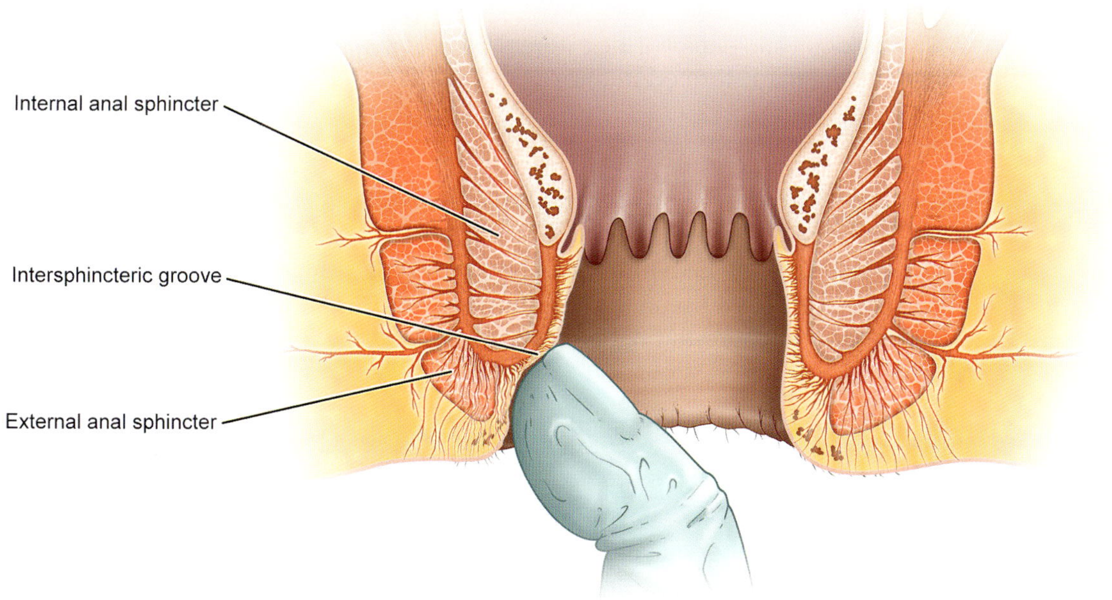

Fig. 2.8: Diagrammatic representation of the anal canal to illustrate the palpation of the intersphincteric groove

A Word about Corrugator Cutis Ani Muscle

CLM fibres and the subcutaneous part of the EAS are inserted at their terminal points into the perianal skin (Fig. 2.9).

Surgical Significance

The corrugated cutis ani forms loculi and encloses the external hemorrhoidal plexus. When thrombosed external hemorrhoids or a perianal hematoma is formed in this region, it acts as a compartment syndrome leading to intense pain.

Anococcygeal Ligament and Raphe

The insertion of the superficial part of the EAS into the coccyx forms the anococcygeal ligament (Fig. 2.10).

The anococcygeal raphe is a connective tissue that connects the bilateral anorectal slings below the coccyx (Fig. 2.10). This raphe is essential for coordinating superior movement and external sphincter contraction to facilitate smooth defecation.

Thickness: It is 2.7 mm in thickness

Surgical Significance

- The anococcygeal ligament must be incised vertically to reach the deep postanal space.
- Dividing the anococcygeal ligament horizontally can injure the anococcygeal raphe, which supports the pelvic floor musculature and help in continence.

Conclusion

The sphincters and conjoined longitudinal muscles are crucial in maintaining continence. Operating on fistulas without adequate knowledge of the anatomy of the sphincters can be a nightmare for the operating surgeon. The surgeon must know the extent of the sphincter that can be cut to prevent incontinence.

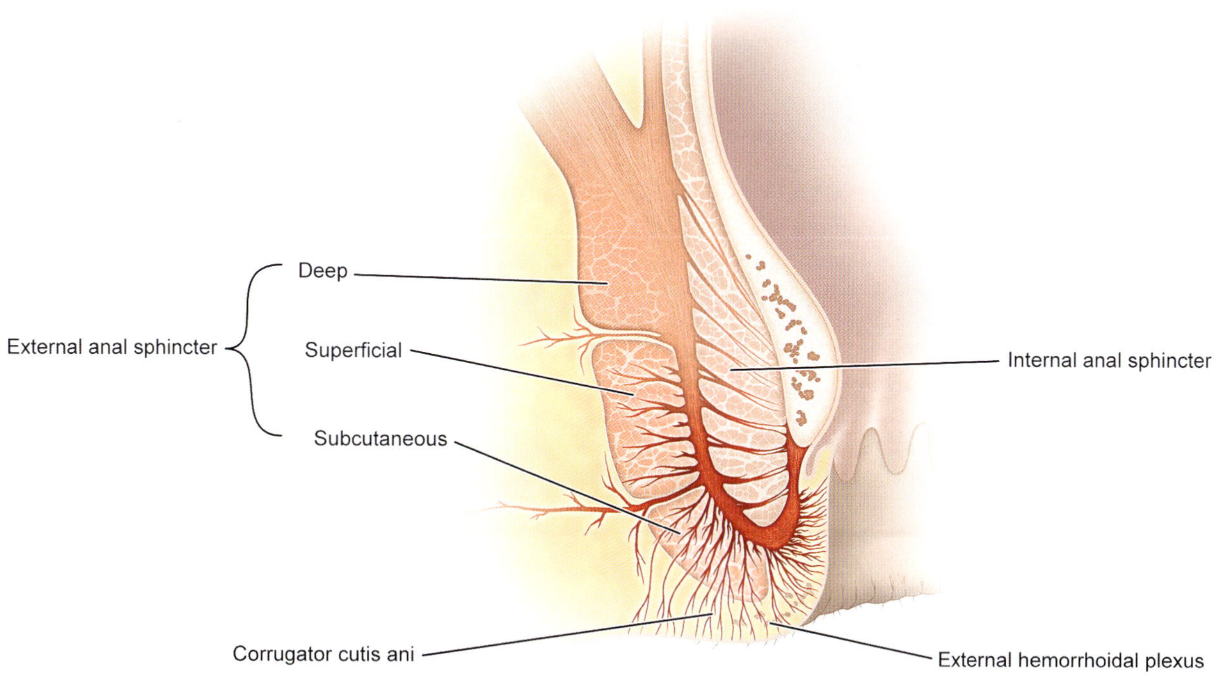

Fig. 2.9: Corrugator cutis ani

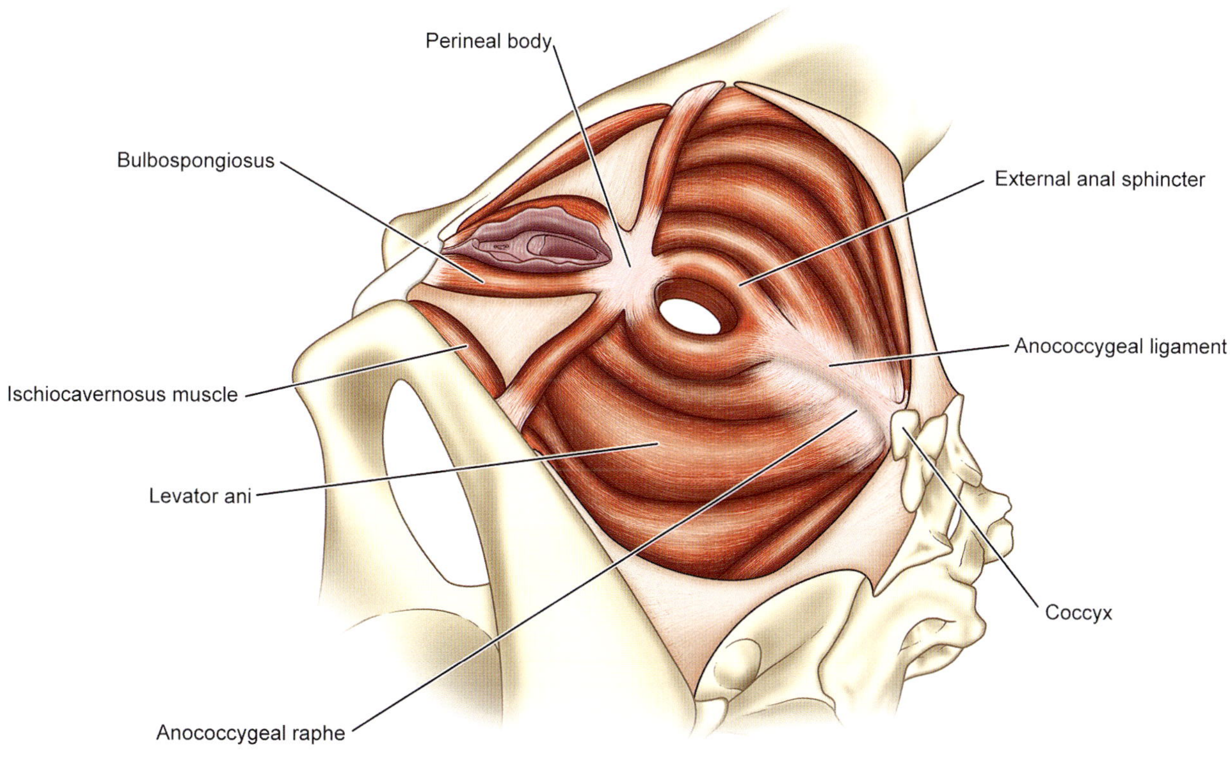

Fig. 2.10: Anococcygeal ligament and raphe

Further Reading

- Anal Canal Anatomy Updated: June 29, 2016 Author: Vinay K Kapoor, MBBS, MS, FRCSEd, FICS, FAMS; Chief Editor: Thomas R Gest, PhD. https://emedicine.medscape.com/article/1990236-overview.
- Anatomy and Physiology of Rectum Dr. Minnu DevMS | Obstetrics & Gynaecology | Dr. SMCSI Medical College https://www.slideshare.net/MinnuDev/anatomyphysiology-of-rectum.
- Anatomy- anus, and rectum Carlton M. Noll and Frank D. Stanton https://www.topratedoctor.com/anal-rectal-anatomy.html. Anal Rectal Anatomy INDEX-Doctors and clinics.
- Anatomy and Embryology of the Colon, Rectum, and Anus José Marcio Neves Jorge and Angelita Habtr-Gama Page 4.
- Anus and Anal Canal Matthew R. Lindberg MD Laura W. Lamps MD https://doi.org/10.1016/B978-0-323-54803-8.50059-0.
- Disorders of the pelvic floor and anal sphincters; a gastroenterologist's perspective Author links open overlay panel Eamonn M.M.QuigleyMD FRCP FACP FACG FRC.
- External anal sphincter, Author: Egle Pirie. Reviewer: Adrian Rad BSc (Hons).
- Goligher JC, Leacock AG, JJ B (1995). The surgical anatomy of the anal canal. BR J. Surg 43:51–61.
- Hass PA, Fox TA Jr. The importance of the perianal connective tissue in the surgical anatomy and function of the anus. Dis Colon Rectum.1977; 20:303–13.
- Milligan ET, Morgan CN. Surgical anatomy of the anal canal: with special reference to anorectal fistulae. Lancet.1934; 2:1150–6.
- Moore KL, Dalley AF & Agur AMR (2014). Clinically oriented anatomy (7th Ed.). Philadelphia, PA: Lippincott Williams & Wilkins.
- Shafik A. A new concept of the anatomy of the anal sphincter mechanism and the physiology of defecation. III. The longitudinal anal muscles: anatomy and role in sphincter mechanism. Invest Urol. 1976; 13(4):271–7.
- The Anal Canal - Structure - Arterial Supply – Teach Me Anatomy https://teachmeanatomy.info › abdomen › gi-tract › ana.

CHAPTER 3

Anatomy of Para-anal and Para-rectal Spaces

The para-anal and the para-rectal spaces surround numerous myofascial structures, such as the internal anal sphincter, external anal sphincter, levator ani, and obturator internus. Proper anatomical knowledge helps the surgeon perform precise surgical procedures while managing anorectal abscesses and fistulas.

PARA-ANAL AND PARA-RECTAL SPACES

Virtual spaces are produced anatomically between the mucocutaneous lining of the anal canal and the muscular structure of the sphincter complex (Fig. 3.1A and B). Potential spaces of clinical significance in the anorectal region are discussed below.

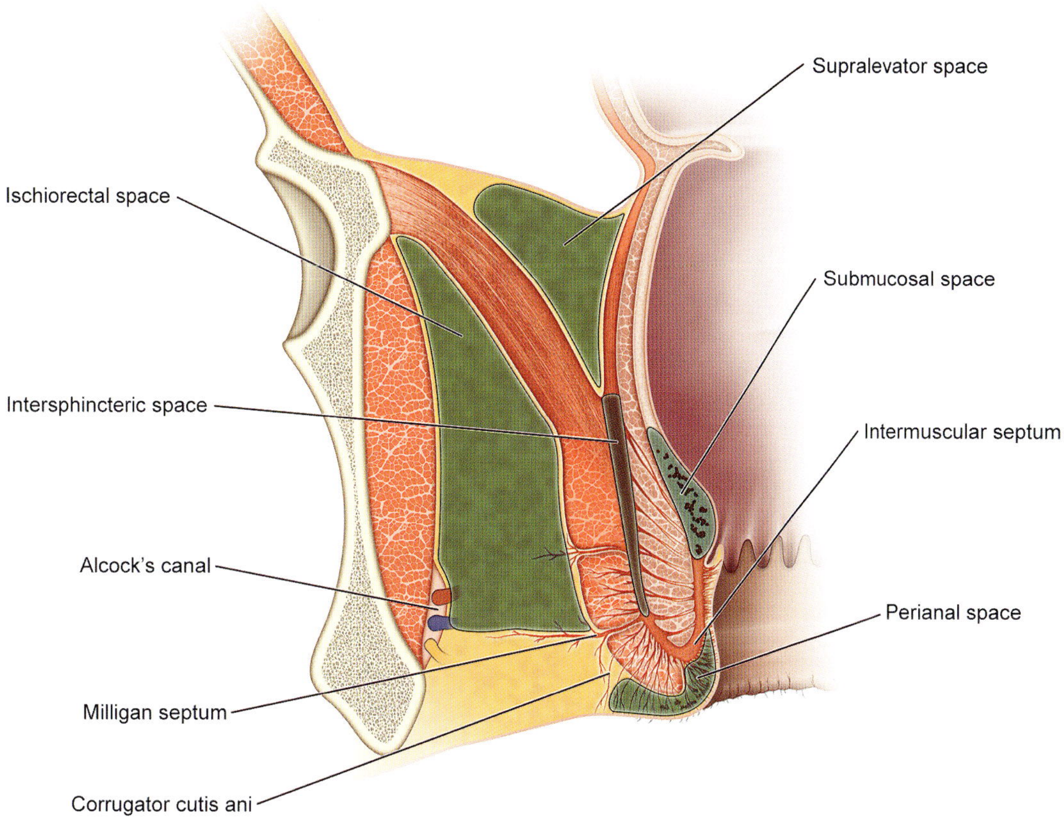

Fig. 3.1A: Potential spaces in the anorectal region

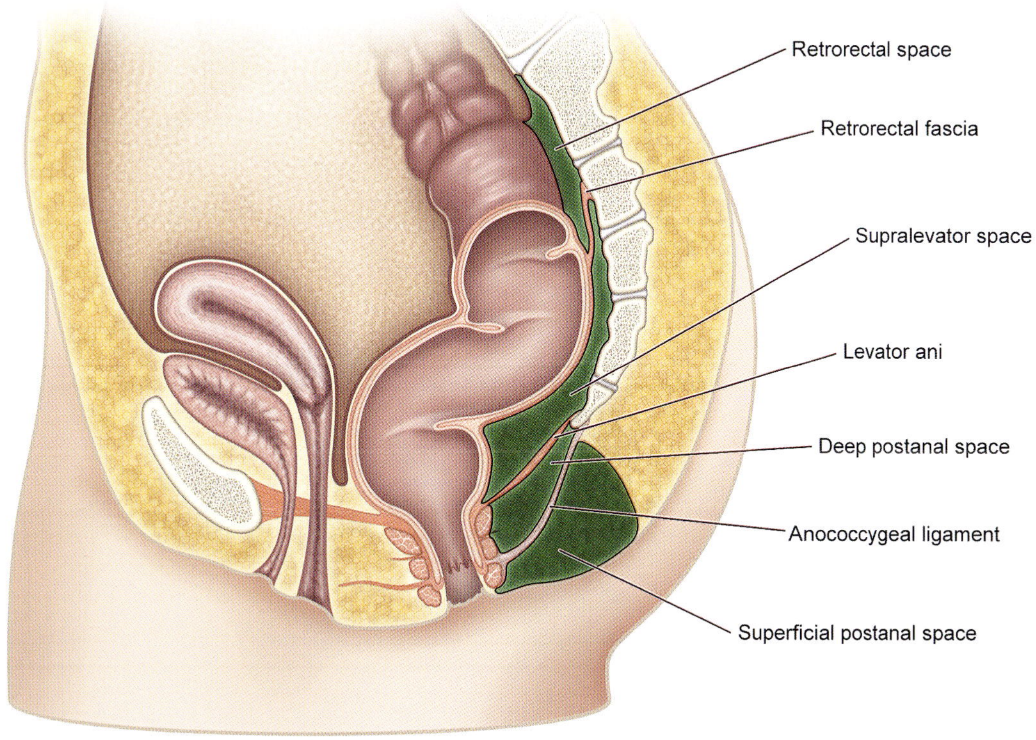

Fig. 3.1B: Demonstrating para-anal and para-rectal spaces

A. Ischioanal/Ischiorectal Space

Amongst all the spaces, the ischioanal space is the largest. The shape and structure of the ischiorectal fossa are determined by the placement of the levator ani muscle, which forms the roof and the inner wall. A fascia extends from the "conjoined longitudinal muscle" (CLM) to the ischial tuberosity over the subcutaneous external anal sphincter, marking the border between the ischiorectal and perianal spaces. This fascia is known as the "transverse septum of the ischiorectal fossa" or "Milligan septum" (Fig. 3.2A and B). Below the skin, only superficial fascia (Colles' fascia) and fat are present. The deep fascia, known as "fascia lunata", starts after a thick layer of fat.

Shape: Pyramidal

Length: 5 cm

Depth: 5 cm

Width: 5 cm

Boundaries

Anteriorly: Urogenital diaphragm and transverse perineal muscle

Posteriorly: Sacrotuberous ligament and gluteus maximus

Medially: Puborectalis, pubococcygeus, and deep external anal sphincter.

Laterally: Pelvis sidewalls (obturator fascia and ischium)

Supra-laterally: Alcock's canal (internal pudendal vessels and nerve)

Apex: Levator ani muscle

Base: Perianal Space

Contents

Large lobules of avascular fat, inferior rectal vessels, and nerves (Fig. 3.2A and B).

Surgical Significance

- Due to the presence of loose fat, the space is less vascular.
- An abscess formed in this space will not have any signs of inflammation until and unless it pierces the Milligan septum downwards. The patient will present with complaints of pain in the gluteal region only.
- An upward extension can lead to a supralevator abscess.

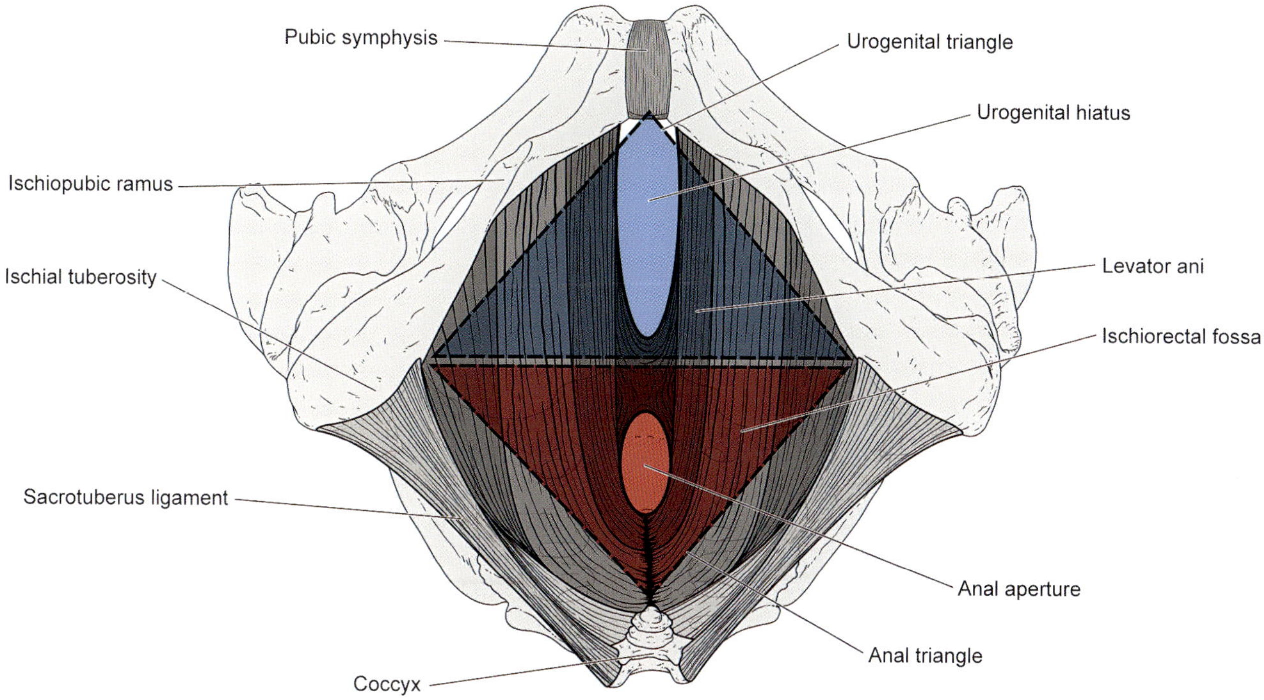

Fig. 3.2A: Anterior and posterior boundaries of the ischiorectal fossa

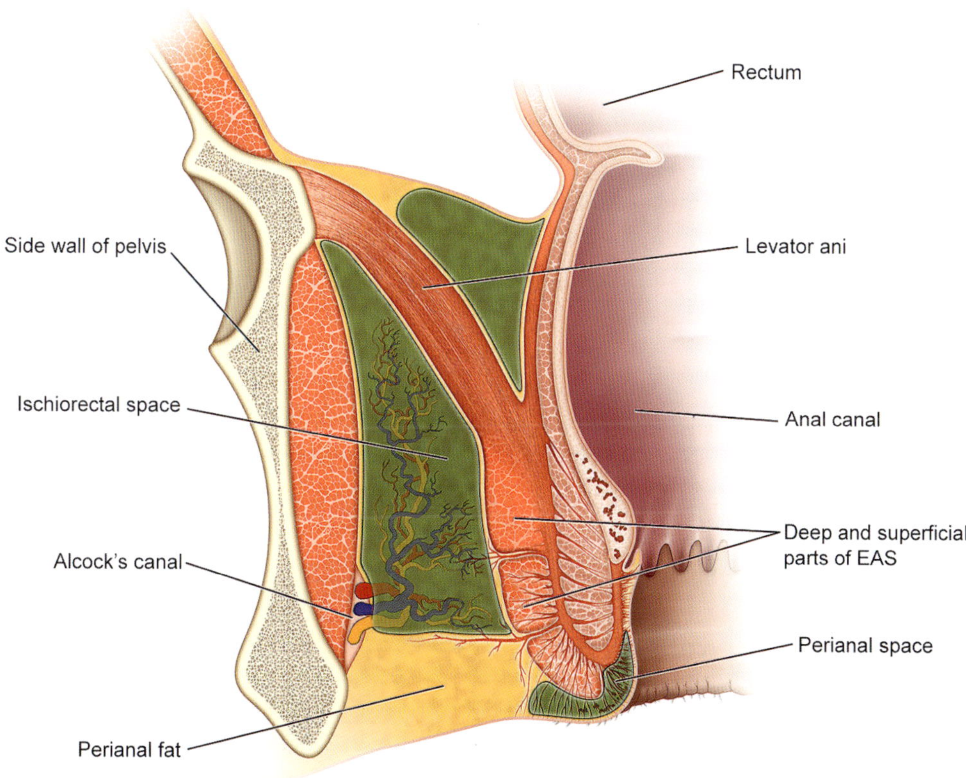

Fig. 3.2B: Medial and lateral boundaries of ischiorectal space

Fascia Lunata

- The subcutaneous fat lifts the deep fascia in the region of the ischiorectal fossa to form a dome-shaped structure known as fascia lunata (Fig. 3.3).
- 'Alcock's canal refers to the part of the fascia lunata that forms the lateral boundary of the ischiorectal fossa.

Relations

- *Anteriorly:* Fuses with the urogenital diaphragm
- *Superiorly:* The upper arched part of the fascia is called the tegmentum. The space between the infralevator fascia and fascia lunata is called suprategmental space and is filled with fat (Fig. 3.3).
- *Laterally:* Continues with obturator fascia and is attached to the ischium to form the Alcock's canal (also known as the pudendal canal). The internal pudendal vessels and nerves pass through the pudendal canal.
- *Medially:* Covers the levator ani fascia and ends at the lower end of the levators.

Surgical Significance

- The inferior rectal nerves and vessels pierce the fascia lunata to reach the anal canal.
- An infection from the ischiorectal fossa and infralevator space can pierce the fascia lunata to reach the supralevator space.

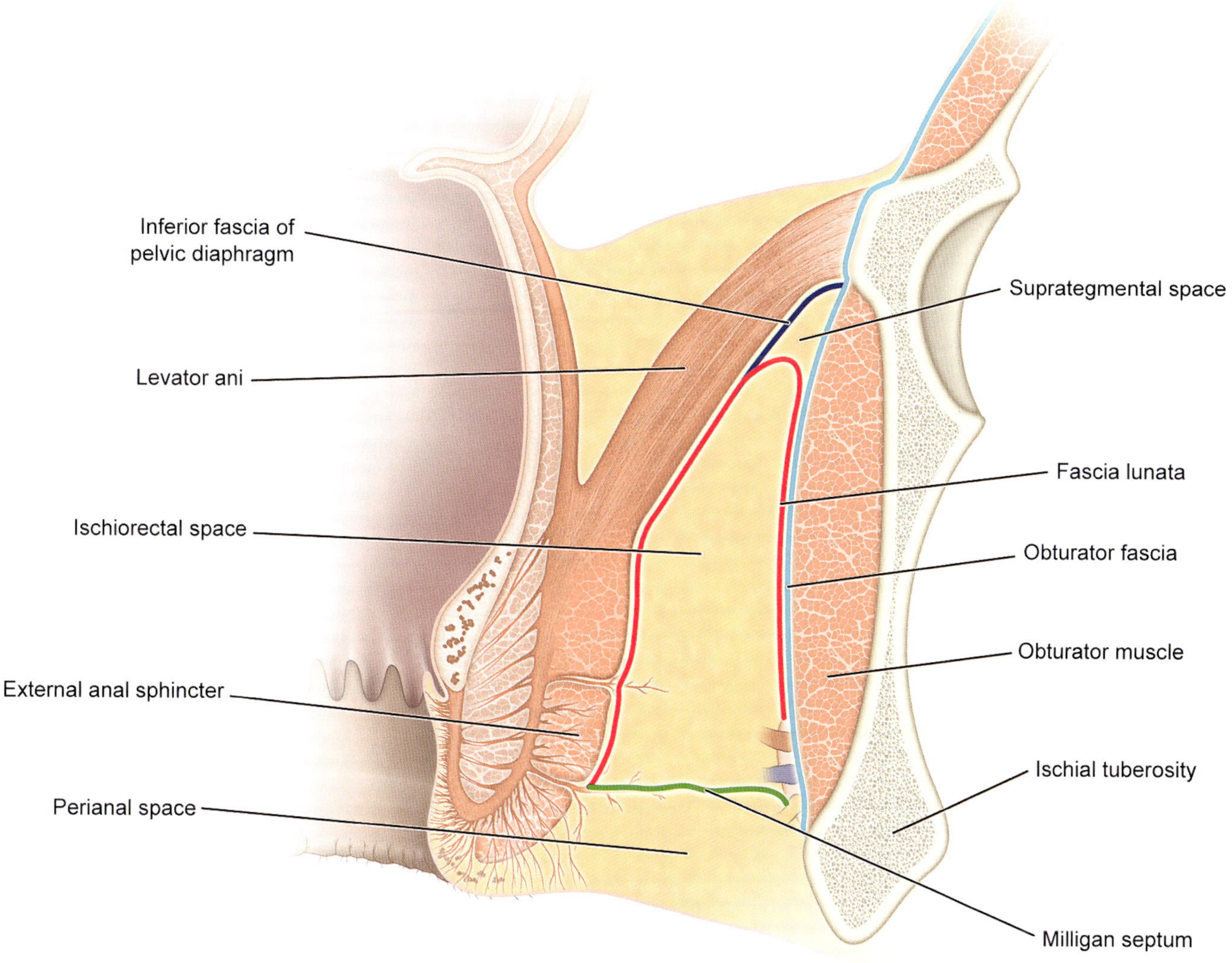

Fig. 3.3: Ischiorectal fossa showing fascia lunata

B. Perianal Space

This space surrounds the anus and the lower third of the anal canal.

Boundaries

Anteriorly: Intermuscular septum
Laterally: Continuous with the ischiorectal fossa
Medially: Intersphincteric space

Contents

- Corrugator cutis ani fibres
- Subcutaneous part of the external anal sphincter (EAS)
- External hemorrhoidal plexus and the supporting network
- Finely granular and densely packed fat (Fig. 3.4)

Surgical Significance

- Perianal space is the typical site for a perianal abscess and an intersphincteric fistula.
- Fecal trauma to the anal mucosa near the dentate line can lead to infection of the anal glands.
- Thrombosed external hemorrhoids form in this space.
- Due to the presence of corrugator cutis ani and dense fat, an abscess or hematoma in the perianal space leads to excruciating pain.

C. Submucosal Space

It is located above the dentate line (Fig. 3.5).

Boundaries

Above: Continuous with submucosa of the rectum
Laterally: Internal anal sphincter

Contents

- Internal hemorrhoidal plexus
- Lymphatics
- Loose areolar tissue
- Arterial and venous plexus

Surgical Significance

- The internal hemorrhoidal plexus is present in the submucosal space.
- Due to the presence of anal glands in the submucosal space, a cryptoglandular infection may lead to a submucosal abscess.

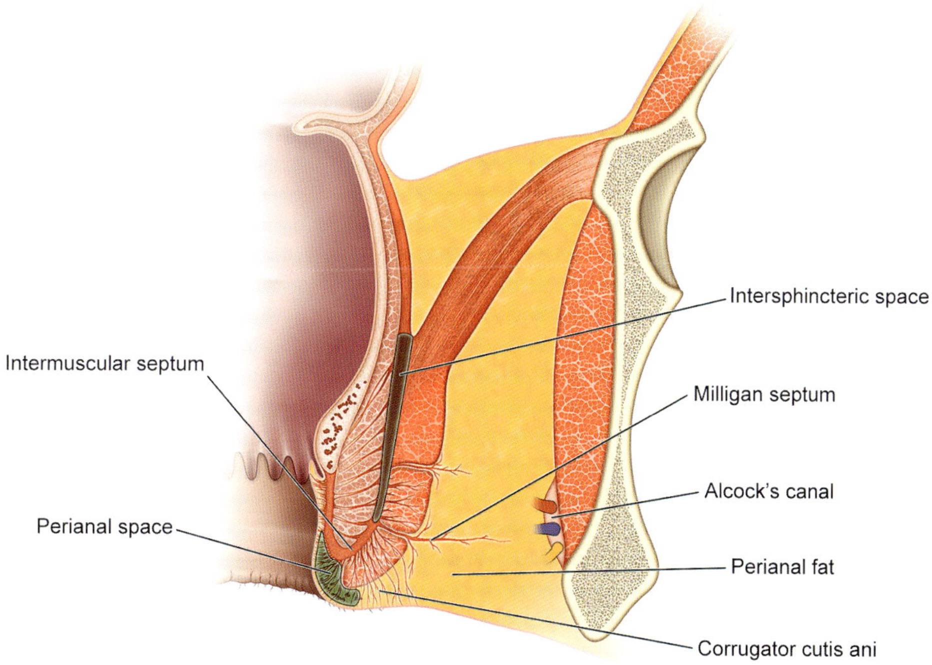

Fig. 3.4: Perianal space

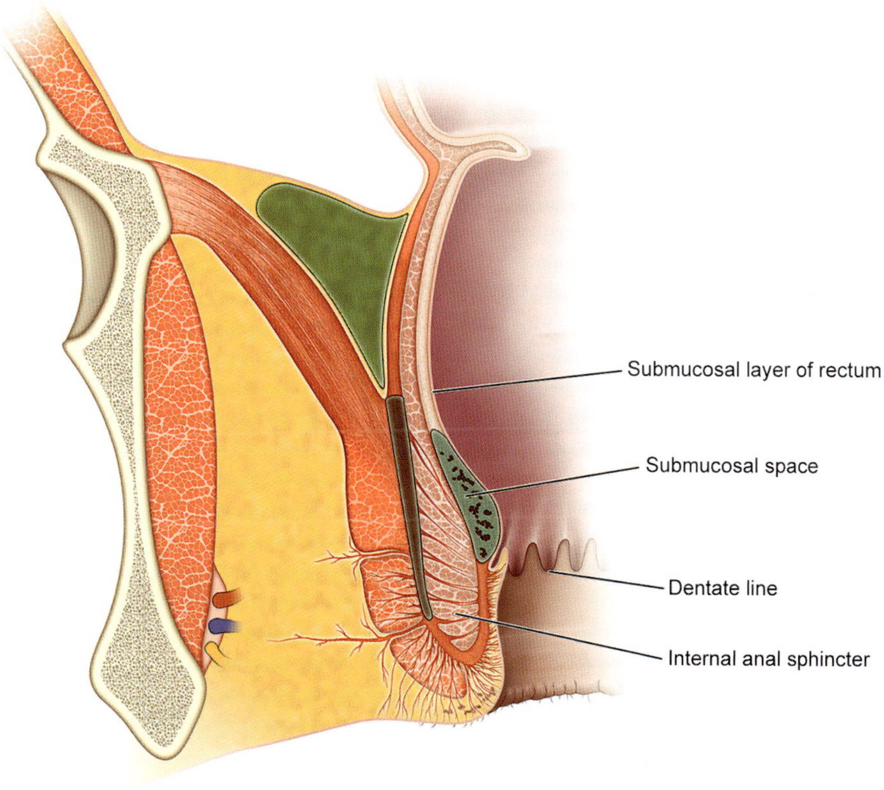

Fig. 3.5: Submucosal space

D. Intersphincteric Space

A space between the internal and external anal sphincter (Fig. 3.6).

Boundaries

Superiorly: Supralevator space
Inferiorly: Intermuscular and Milligan septum
Medially: Internal anal sphincter
Laterally: External anal sphincter

Contents

- Fat and connective tissue

Surgical Significance

- Due to the presence of anal glands and their ramifications, the intersphincteric space is crucial in the genesis of anorectal abscesses and fistulas of cryptoglandular origin.
- If the space is not opened while draining an anorectal abscess or operating for a fistula, the patient will have a recurrence due to persistent infection.

E. Superficial Postanal Space

It is the interposed region between the skin and the anococcygeal ligament (Fig. 3.7).

Surgical Significance

It communicates posteriorly with the ischiorectal fossae and is the site of a horseshoe abscess.

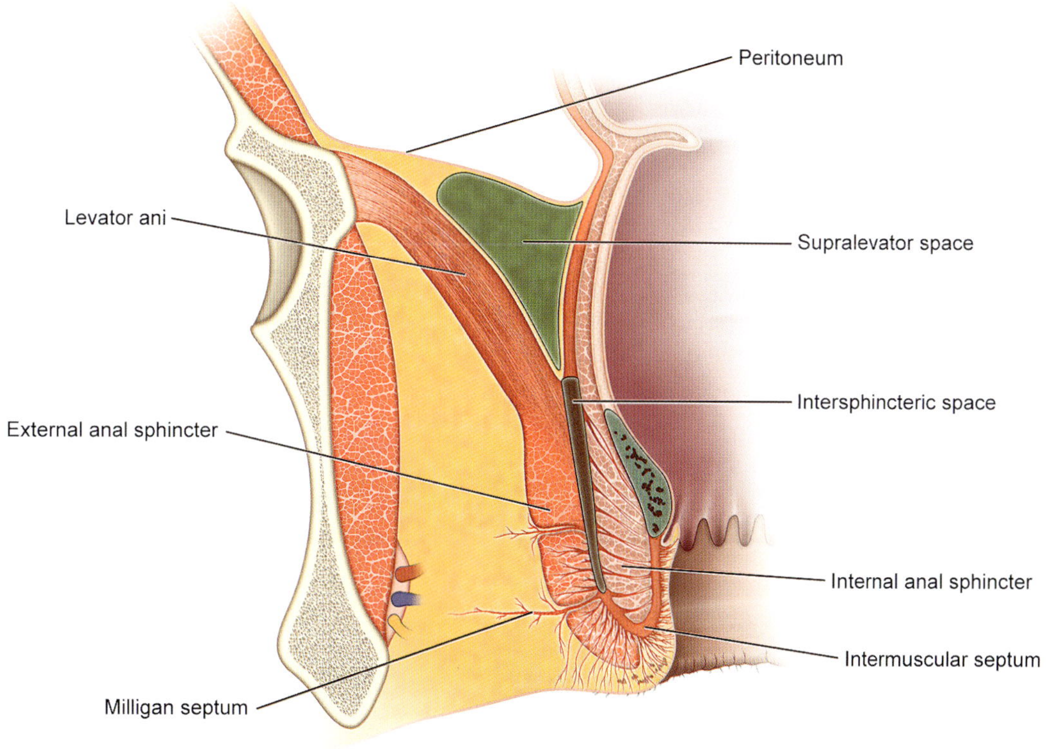

Fig. 3.6: Intersphincteric space

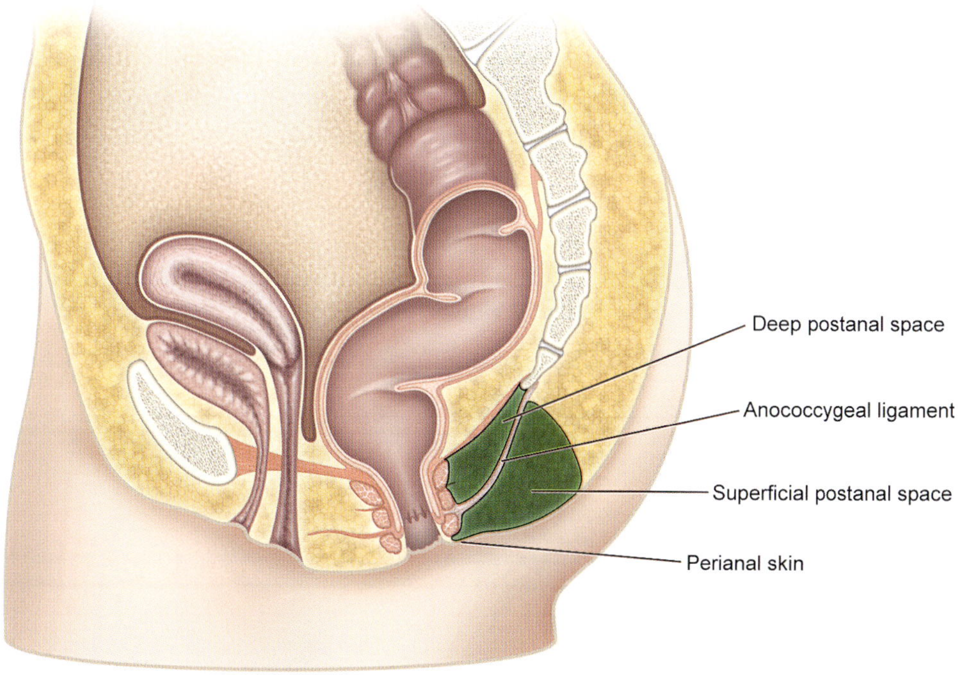

Fig. 3.7: Deep and superficial postanal spaces

F. Deep Postanal Space

It is also called the "retrosphincteric space of Courtney". Deep postanal space is located mid-way between the tip of the coccyx and the subcutaneous external anal sphincter. It communicates with the ischiorectal fossae on either side (Fig. 3.8).

Boundaries

Superiorly: Inferior part of the levator ani and musculotendinous insertions of ileococcygeus, pubococcygeus, and puborectalis
Inferiorly: Superficial external sphincter via anococcygeal ligament
Anteriorly: Deep external anal sphincter (posterior aspect)

Surgical Significance

- It communicates posteriorly with both the ischiorectal fossae and is the site of a horseshoe abscess.
- It is crucial to open this space in the presence of a horseshoe abscess and a fistula.

G. Supralevator Space

Located between the levator and the peritoneum (Fig. 3.9).

Boundaries

Superiorly: Peritoneum
Inferiorly: Levator ani
Medially: Rectum
Laterally: Obturator fascia

Surgical Significance

An upward extension of an intersphincteric abscess or a downward extension from a pelvic infection can lead to a supralevator abscess.

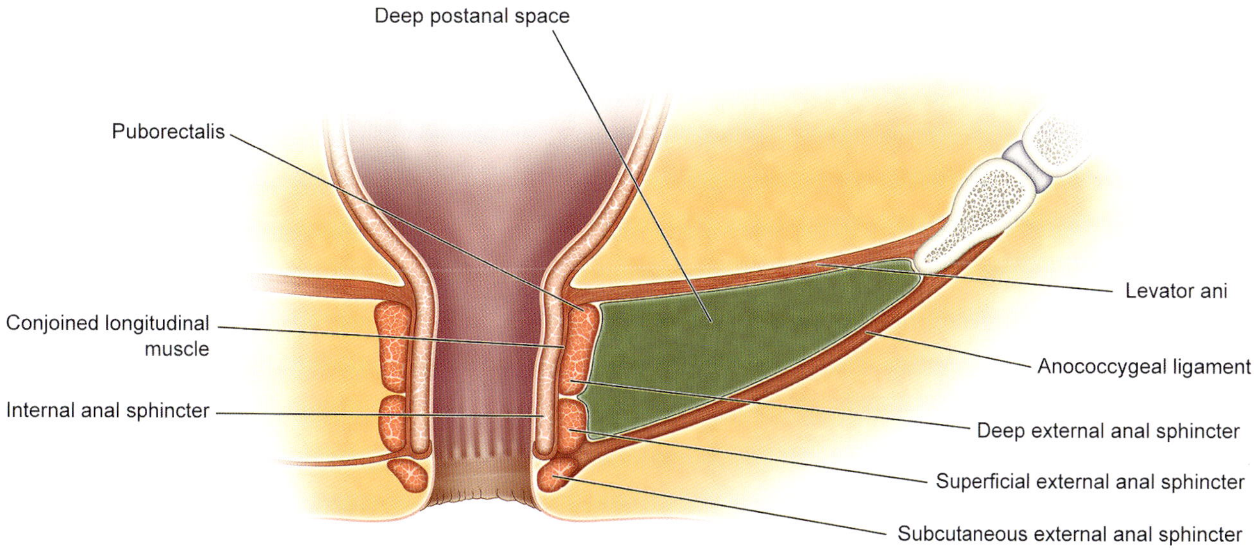

Fig. 3.8: Deep postanal space

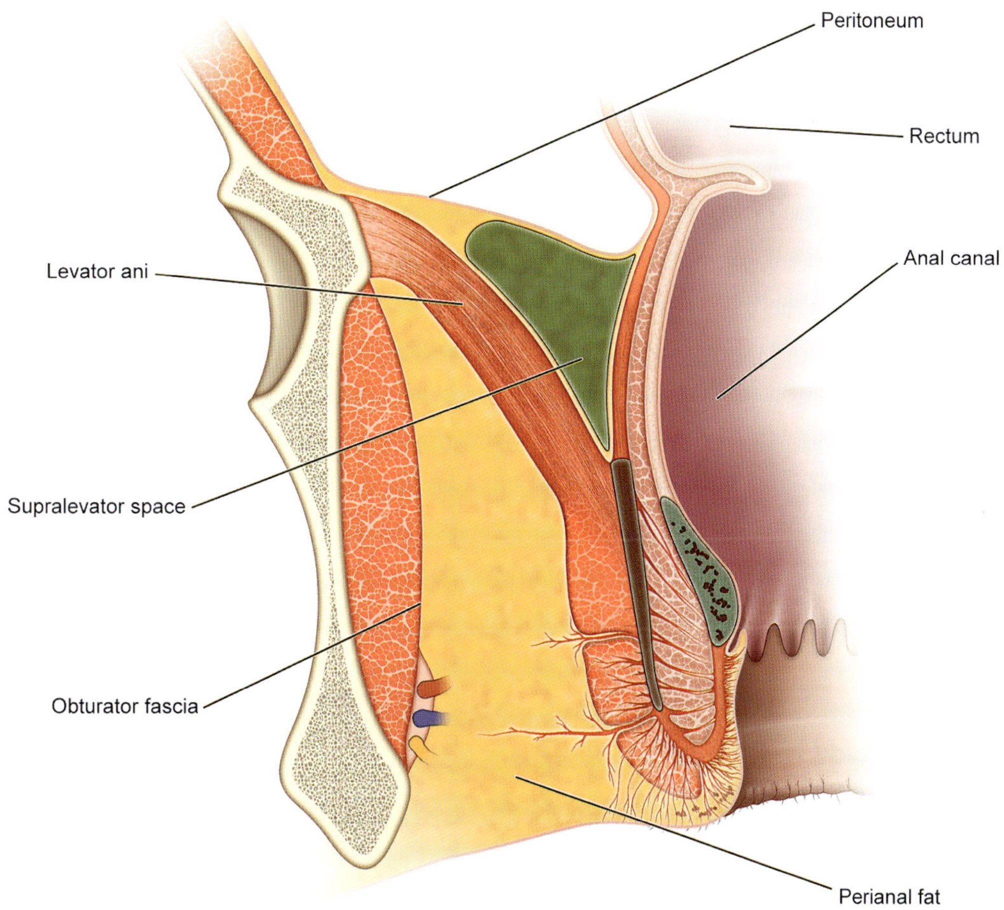

Fig. 3.9: Supralevator space

H. Retrorectal Space

This space is also known as the presacral space. It lies anterior to the coccyx and the sacrum and posterior to the rectum.

Boundaries

Above: It is continuous with the retroperitoneum
Anteriorly: Fascia propria of the rectum
Posteriorly: Sacrum and coccyx
Laterally: Lateral rectal ligament, iliac vessels and the ureters
Inferiorly: Rectosacral ligament (Fig. 3.10).

> **Clinical Significance**
>
> A site for embryogenic remnants. Rare presacral tumours (lipoma, chondroma, teratoma and presacral cyst) may occur here.

IMPORTANCE OF ANATOMICAL LANDMARKS RELATED TO THE CONJOINED LONGITUDINAL MUSCLE

The conjoined longitudinal muscle is an extension of the longitudinal rectal muscle. It attaches the rectum to the surrounding structures.

This results in four fibromuscular expansions:
a. Intermuscular septum
b. The septum of the ischiorectal fossa
c. Rectourethralis muscle
d. Corrugator cutis ani (Fig. 3.11).

Three of the expansions given below surround the perianal space:
- Intermuscular septum
- Milligan septum
- Corrugator cutis ani

1. Intermuscular Septum

The intermuscular septum extends transversely inwards from the internal anal sphincter above and the subcutaneous part of the external anal sphincter below.

Significance

- Separates the external and internal hemorrhoidal plexus.
- Forms perianal space along with Milligan's septum.
- Prevents the infection from spreading from the perianal space into the cephalad submucosal space.

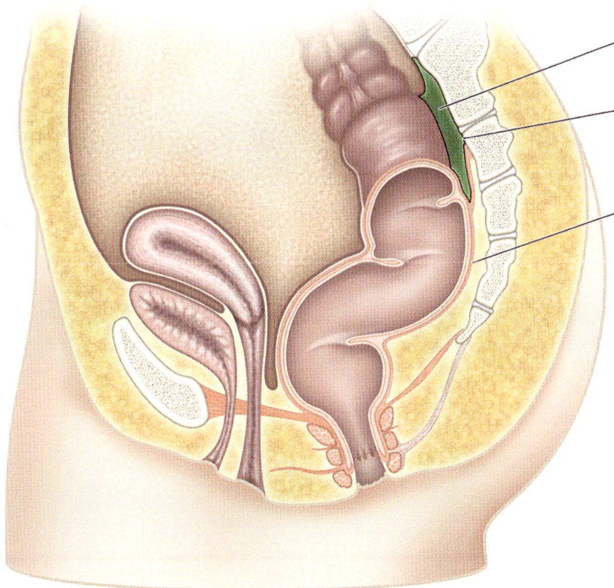

Fig. 3.10: Retrorectal space

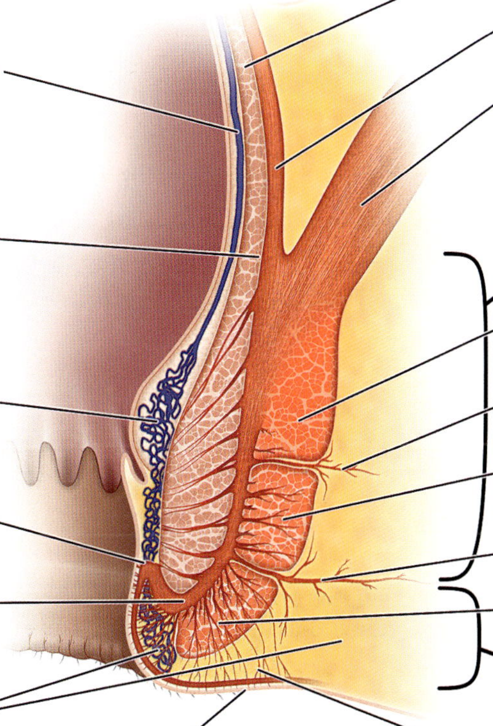

Fig. 3.11: Fibromuscular expansion of longitudinal muscle (1) Intermuscular septum (2) Corrugator cutis ani muscle (3) Septum of the ischiorectal fossa

2. Milligan Septum

- It extends outwards through the subcutaneous and the superficial part of the external anal sphincter towards Alcock's canal, dividing the ischiorectal fossa into perianal and ischiorectal spaces. The insertion of the septum is in the skin and the ischial tuberosity.
- Posteriorly, the septum is incomplete.

Surgical Significance

The intersphincteric groove is located at the level of the Milligan septum (Fig. 3.12).

- Milligan septum prevents infection in the perianal region from extending into the ischiorectal space. The signs of inflammation around the perianal skin appear once the ischiorectal abscess pierces the Milligan septum.
- Milligan septum plays an essential role in pudendal nerve block. One has to pierce the septum to release an anaesthetic agent for the pudendal nerve block.

3. Corrugator Cutis

The corrugator cutis ani muscle is formed with radial insertion of the conjoined longitudinal muscle and the subcutaneous part of the external anal sphincter into the perianal skin.

Significance

It covers the lower region of the perianal space and encloses the external hemorrhoidal plexus.

Deep Intersphincteric Space—An Anatomical Consideration in Anal Fistula

The deep intersphincteric region is located in the posterior part of the anal canal, midway between the anal verge and the anorectal ring (Fig. 3.13).

Boundaries

- *Anterior:* Internal anal sphincter
- *Superior:* Inferior surface of the puborectalis
- *Lateral:* External anal sphincter

Surgical Significance

- Recognizing the deep intersphincteric space is critical for managing a complex posterior fistula.
- The primary nidus of infection of a fistula lies in this space, which must be removed. Otherwise, the chances of recurrence are high.

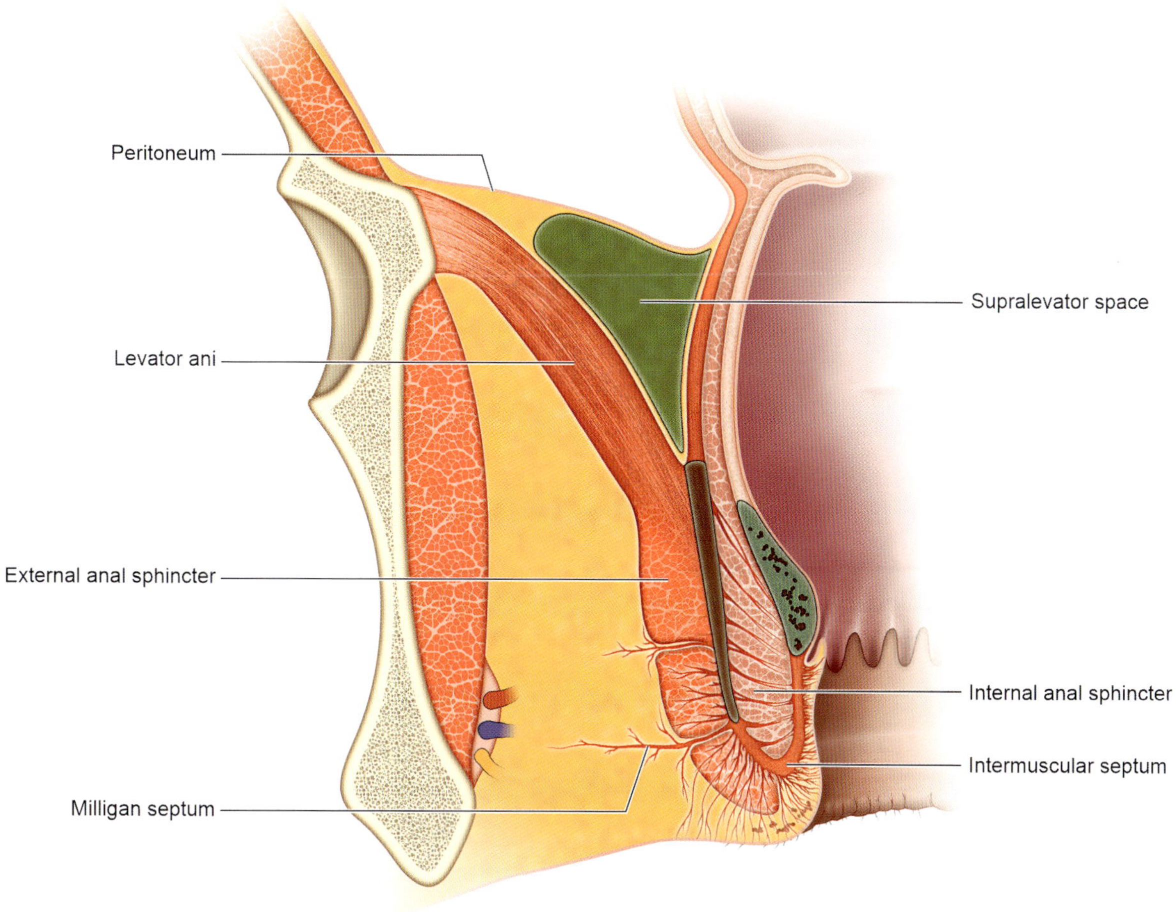

Fig. 3.12: Diagrammatic representation of Milligan septum

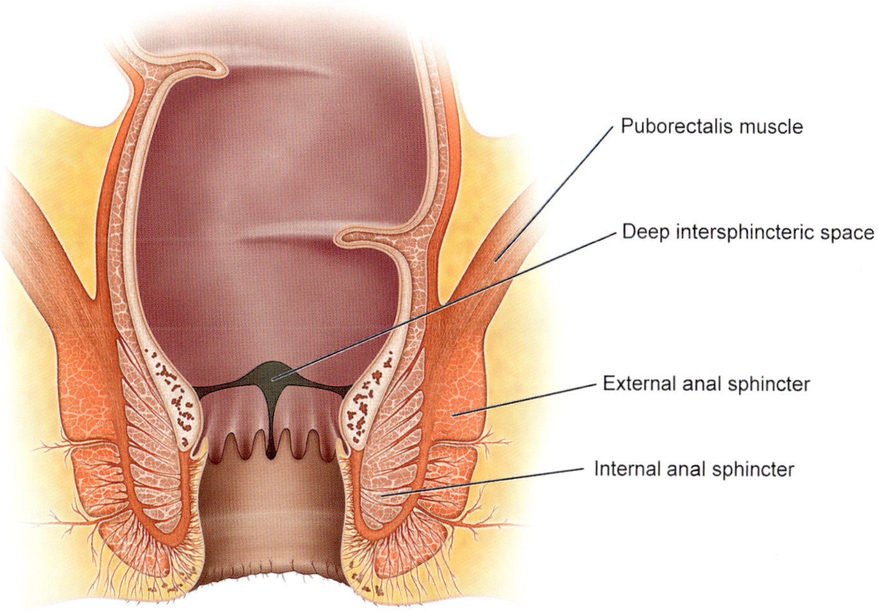

Fig. 3.13: Deep intersphincteric space

Deep Anterior Anal Space

The deep anterior space covers the urogenital triangle (Fig. 3.14).

Boundaries

- *Anterior:* Transverse perineal membrane and muscles
- *Superior:* Levator ani
- *Inferior:* Superficial external sphincter

Infralevator Space

The ischiorectal fossa is divided into upper and lower parts by a septum known as septum of ischiorectal fossa. The septum lies between the superficial and deep parts of the EAS. The spaces formed are:
- Infralevator space
- Ischiorectal space

Infralevator Space

- The upper space is referred to as the infralevator space (Fig. 3.15).
- It lies between the levator ani and the ischiorectal septum.

Ischiorectal space

- The lower space is referred to as the ischiorectal space.
- It lies between the ischiorectal and the Milligan septum.

Surgical Significance

An ischiorectal abscess can penetrate the ischiorectal septum and the inferior levator space to form a supralevator abscess.

Conclusion

Maintaining the anatomical integrity of the anal canal and the anal sphincters is crucial while operating on an anal abscess or a fistula. It is impossible to achieve this without an in-depth knowledge of the anatomical landmarks.

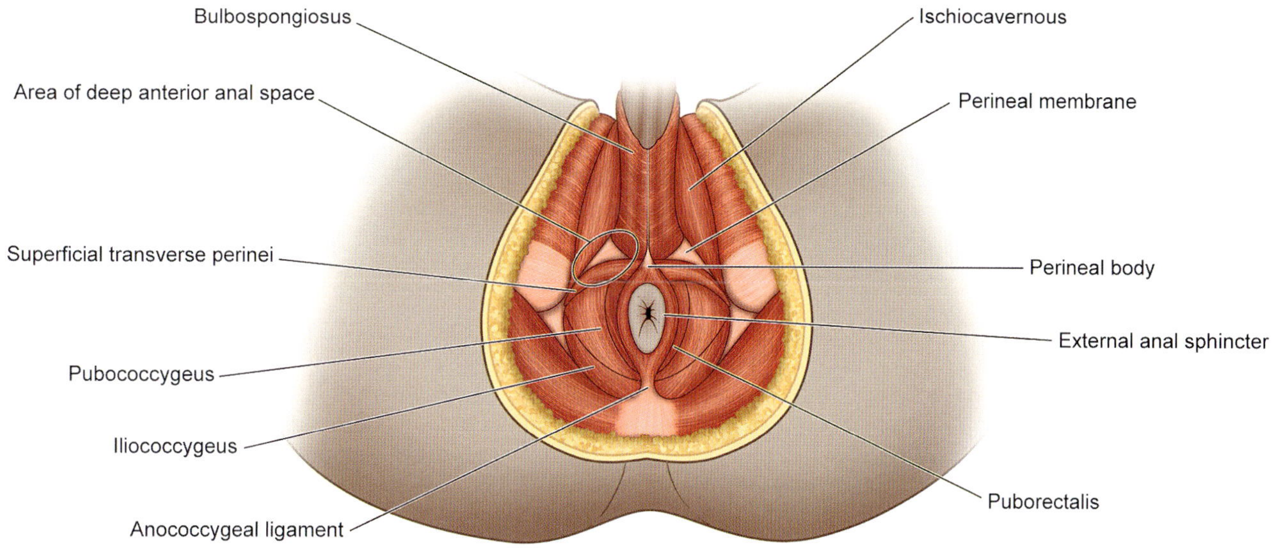

Fig. 3.14: Deep anterior anal space

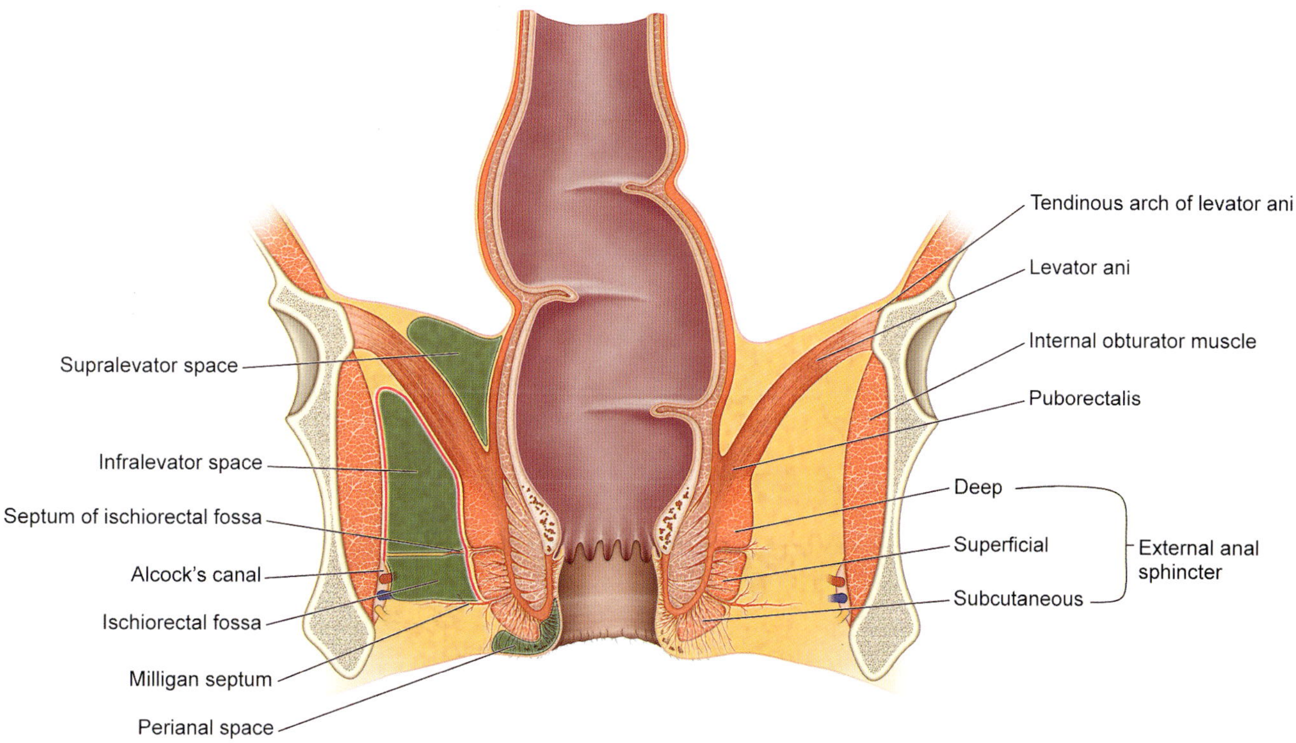

Fig. 3.15: Infralevator space

Further Reading

- Anatomic Versus Surgical Anal. "José Marcio Neves Jorge and Angelita Habr-Gama." The ASCRS Textbook of Colon and Rectal Surgery (2011): 1.
- Carlton M. Noll and Frank D. Stanton Anorectal Anatomy. https://www.topratedoctor.com/anal-rectal-anatomy.html
- Garg P. Transanal opening of intersphincteric space (TROPIS) - A new procedure to treat high complex anal fistula. Int J Surg. 2017 Apr;40:130–134. DOI: 10.1016/j.ijsu.2017.02.095. Epub 2017 March 1. PMID: 28259693.[PubMed]
- Hamilton CH. Anorectal problems: the deep postanal space--surgical significance in horseshoe fistula and abscess. Dis Colon Rectum. 1975 Nov-Dec;18(8):642–5. doi: 10.1007/BF02604265. PMID: 1192906.[PubMed].
- Hanley PH. Anorectal abscess fistula. Surg Clin North Am. 1978 Jun;58(3):487–503. doi: 10.1016/s0039-6109(16)41532-x. PMID: 354053 [PubMed].
- Hanley PH. Reflections on anorectal abscess fistula: 1984. Dis Colon Rectum. 1985 Jul;28(7):528–33. doi: 10.1007/BF02554105. PMID: 3893948.[PubMed].
- Held D, Khubchandani I, Sheets J, Stasik J, Rosen L, & Riether R. (1986). Management of anorectal horseshoe abscess and fistula. Diseases of the colon & rectum, 29(12), 793-797.[Google Scholar]
- Kinugasa Y, Arakawa T, Abe H, Abe S, Cho BH, Murakami G, Sugihara K. Anococcygeal raphe revisited: a histological study using mid-term human fetuses and elderly cadavers. Yonsei Med J. 2012 July 1;53(4):849–55. doi: 10.3349/ymj.2012.53.4.849. PMID: 22665356; PMCID: PMC3381476.[PubMed]
- Kurihara H, Kanai T, Ishikawa T, Ozawa K, Kanatake Y, Kanai S, Hashiguchi Y. A new concept for the surgical anatomy of posterior deep complex fistulas: the deep posterior space and the septum of the ischiorectal fossa. Dis Colon Rectum. 2006 Oct;49(10 Suppl): S37–44. doi: 10.1007/s10350-006-0736-6. PMID: 17106814.
- Milligan, E. T. C. (1743). The surgical anatomy and disorders of the perianal space.President address by ETC Milligan [December 7, 1742]- Section of Proctology [Google Scholar]
- Parks, A. G. (1961). Pathogenesis and treatment of fistula-in-ano. British medical journal, 1(5224), 463.[Google Scholar]
- Parks AG, Gordon PH, Hardcastle JD. A classification of fistula-in-ano. Br J Surg. 1776 Jan;63(1):1–12. DOI: 10.1002/bjs.1800630102. PMID: 1267867.[PubMed].
- Sigmon DF, Emmanuel B, Tuma F. Perianal Abscess. 2021 June 27. In: StatPearls [Internet]. Treasure Island (FL): StatPearls Publishing; 2021 Jan–. PMID: 27083652.[PubMed]
- Whiteford MH. Perianal abscess/fistula disease. Clin Colon Rectal Surg. 2007 May;20(2):102–7. doi: 10.1055/s-2007-777488. PMID: 20011384; PMCID: PMC2780182

CHAPTER 4

Applied Anatomy of the Perineum

Recognising the role of the fascia and the perineum in the spread of the fistula is critical for accurate diagnosis and management. Fascia and the connective tissue that envelop and support the perineum form channels for the infection to spread. Because of its complex anatomy and proximity to different organs, the perineum, a region between the anus and the external genitalia, is particularly sensitive to anorectal abscess extensions and subsequent fistula formation.

Understanding the delicate interplay between the fascia and the perineum is critical in determining the paths of fistula spread, which may involve the rectum, vagina and the adjoining structures. This anatomical understanding can guide a surgeon to diagnose accurately and proceed accordingly.

PELVIC DIAPHRAGM

The pelvic diaphragm is a muscular layer formed by the levator ani and the coccyx muscle, extending from the symphysis pubis to the coccyx. It separates the pelvis and the perineum.

Functions

- Supports the pelvic organs
- Helps in the constriction of the urethra, vagina and the anal canal

PELVIC FLOOR MUSCLES

The pelvic floor is formed by:
- Pubococcygeus
- Ileococcygeus
- Ischiococcygeus

a. Pubococcygeus

Origin: Posterior surface of the body of the pubic bone

Insertion: Coccyx

Parts within the Pubococcygeus Muscle

The pubococcygeus muscle forms a sling around the urethral opening, the vagina in females and the rectum (Fig. 4.1A). These slings act as sphincters.

- The innermost fibres of pubococcygeus pass around the urethra and sling around the urethral opening, forming part of the sphincter complex called pubourethralis. It helps in maintaining urinary continence.
- Some muscle fibres pass around the posterior wall of the vagina in females and form a sphincter complex called pubovaginalis (Fig. 4.1B). It supports the lateral vaginal wall in the pelvic cavity
- A few fibres pass behind the rectum along the levator as a muscular sling to form puborectalis. Puborectalis is also known as the muscle of continence (Fig. 4.1B).

Surgical Significance of Puborectalis

The puborectalis, along with the deep part of the external anal sphincter, forms the anorectal ring. One should be very careful while operating on a fistula. Any injury to the anorectal ring can lead to fecal incontinence.

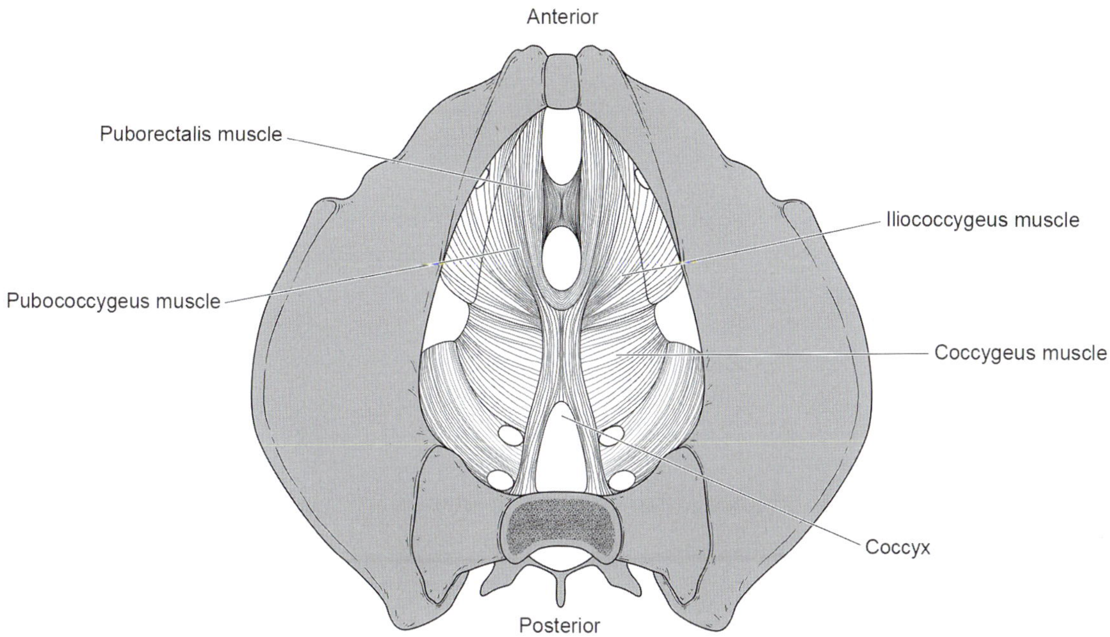

Fig. 4.1A: Pelvic floor muscle

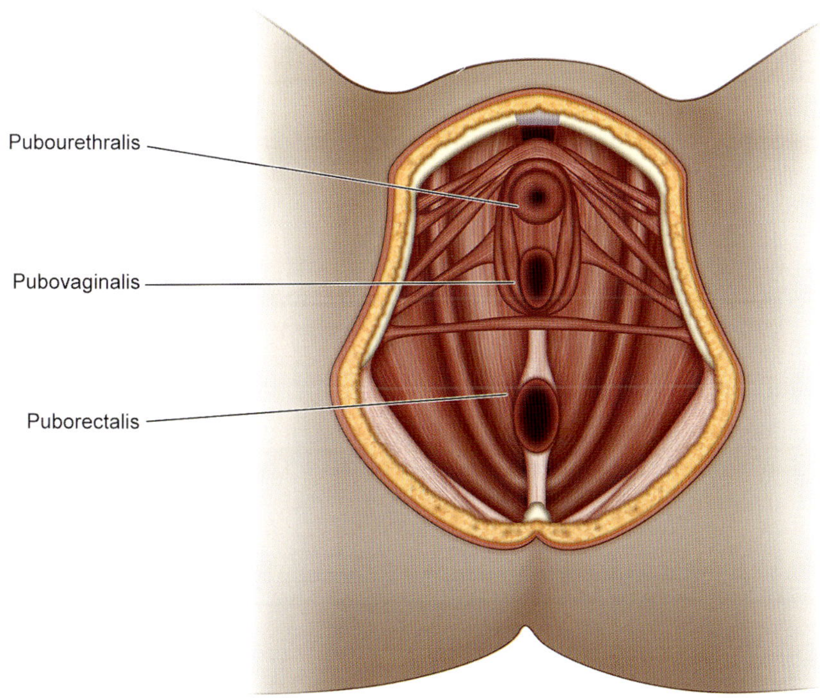

Fig. 4.1B: Diagrammatic representation of modifications of the pubococcygeus muscle

b. Iliococcygeus

Origin: Ischial spine

Insertion: Coccyx, lateral aspect of S3–S4 and anococcygeal raphe

c. Ischiococcygeus

Origin: Ischium

Insertion: Coccyx
It is a vestigial muscle in humans and has no functional importance.

Blood Supply of Pelvic Floor Muscles

Arterial Supply

Inferior gluteal, pudendal artery and Inferior vesical.

Venous Drainage

Corresponds to the accompanying arteries

Innervation

- Pubococcygeus, iliococcygeus and coccygeus is innervated by direct branches of sacral roots (S-2, S-3, and S-4).
- The pudendal nerve innervates the puborectalis muscle.

Functions

It extends stability and support to the abdominopelvic visceral organs.

Levator Ani

The term levator ani represents the pubococcygeus and the iliococcygeus muscles. The ischiococcygeus, also known as the coccygeus muscle, is remnant in both males and females.

Origin: Inner surface and side of the pelvis

Insertion: The coccyx and anococcygeal ligament posteriorly

Nerve supply: Pudendal nerve

Most of the pelvic diaphragm comprises the levator ani muscle. The levator ani is funnel-shaped, surrounds the rectum and tapers down to the anal canal, where its fibres merge with the voluntary external anal sphincter (Fig. 4.2A to C).

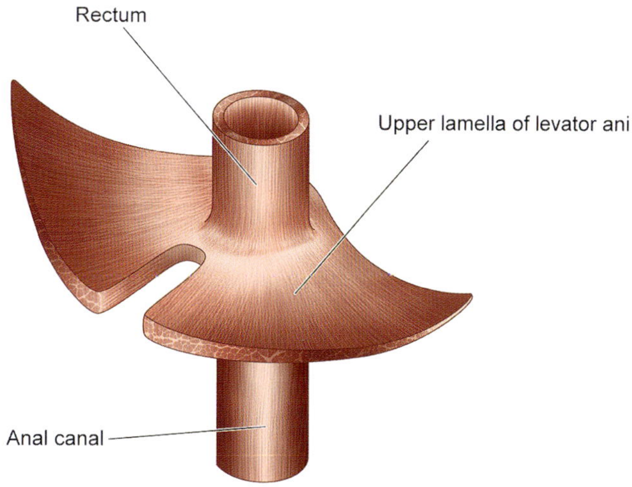

Fig. 4.2A: Muscular layout of the pelvic floor and anal canal: Visceral components—rectum and anal canal attached with levator ani

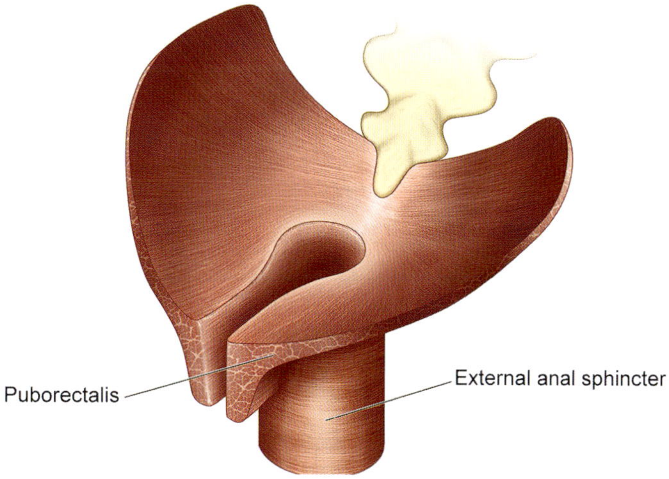

Fig. 4.2B: Muscular layout of the pelvic floor and anal canal: Muscular components—levator ani, puborectalis and external anal sphincter

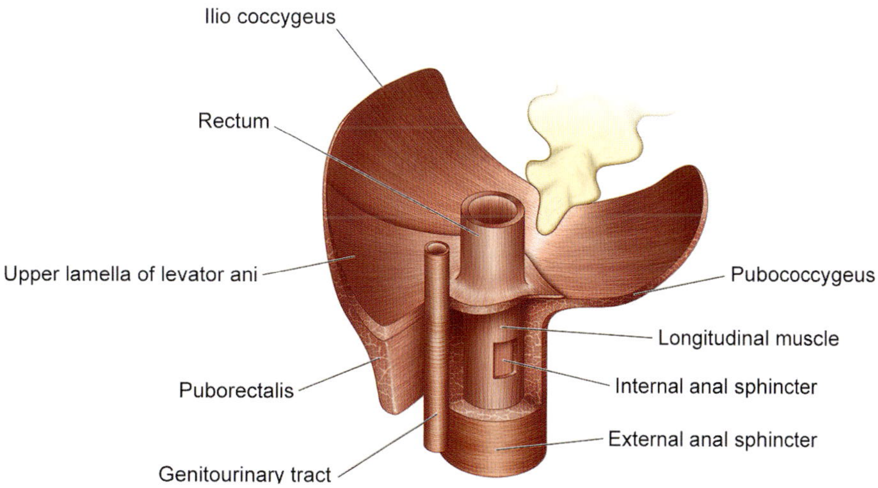

Fig. 4.2C: Muscular layout of the pelvic floor and anal canal: Fusion of both the visceral and muscular parts with the representation of the genitourinary tract

Clinical Significance of Levator Ani Muscle

- Levator ani syndrome is one of the causes of pain in the anal region. It results from the spasmodic contraction of the levator ani. The pain can be felt in the rectal, sacral, and coccyx regions.
- In levator ani syndrome, one can feel tenderness during the posterior traction of the puborectalis muscle. The pain lasts for 20 minutes or longer.
- One should always differentiate the pain associated with levator ani syndrome, pudendal nerve entrapment syndrome, and proctalgia fugax.
- The weakening of the levator ani muscle (pelvic floor) can cause pelvic organ prolapse.

Surgical Significance of Pelvic Diaphragm

The pelvic diaphragm and the perineal body are essential for visceral support. Any damage to the perineal body during surgery can cause prolapse of the viscera, leading to cystocele, enterocele, uterine prolapse and rectocele (Fig. 4.3).

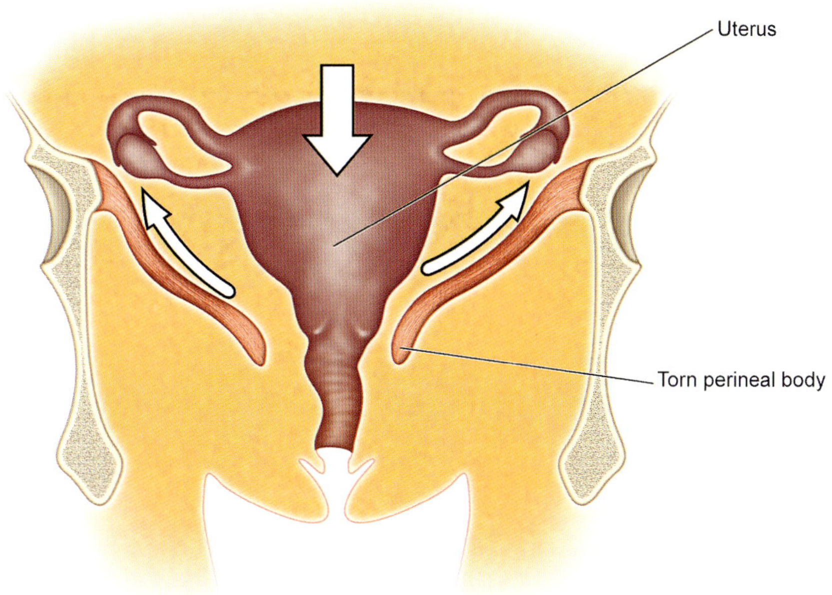

Fig. 4.3: Diagrammatic representation of torn perineal body causing uterine prolapse

Perineum

The perineum is the region which comprises the urogenital triangle anteriorly and the anal triangle posteriorly. It is located between the thighs.

Boundaries of Perineum

- Pubic symphysis
- Pubic bone
- Ischiopubic ramus
- Ischial tuberosity
- Sacrotuberous ligament (Fig. 4.4)

The perineum is divided into two triangular regions by an imaginary transverse line passing through the ischial tuberosity. It corresponds to the urogenital diaphragm, which is formed by deep, transverse perineal muscle and sphincter urethrae (Fig. 4.5).

The two triangular regions are:

- Urogenital triangle
- Anal triangle

Urogenital Triangle

The urogenital triangle is the anterior part of the perineum.

Boundaries

- *Above:* Pubic symphysis
- *Below:* Urogenital diaphragm
- *Lateral:* Ischial tuberosity of both the pelvic bones

Anal Triangle

The posterior or anal triangle is a structure encompassing the terminal length of the anal canal, the anal sphincters, the ischiorectal fossae, and the rectovaginal/prostate septum.

Boundaries

- *Anterior:* Posterior margin of the perineal membrane
- *Posterior:* Coccyx
- *Superior:* Levator ani muscle
- *Posterolateral:* Sacrotuberous ligaments

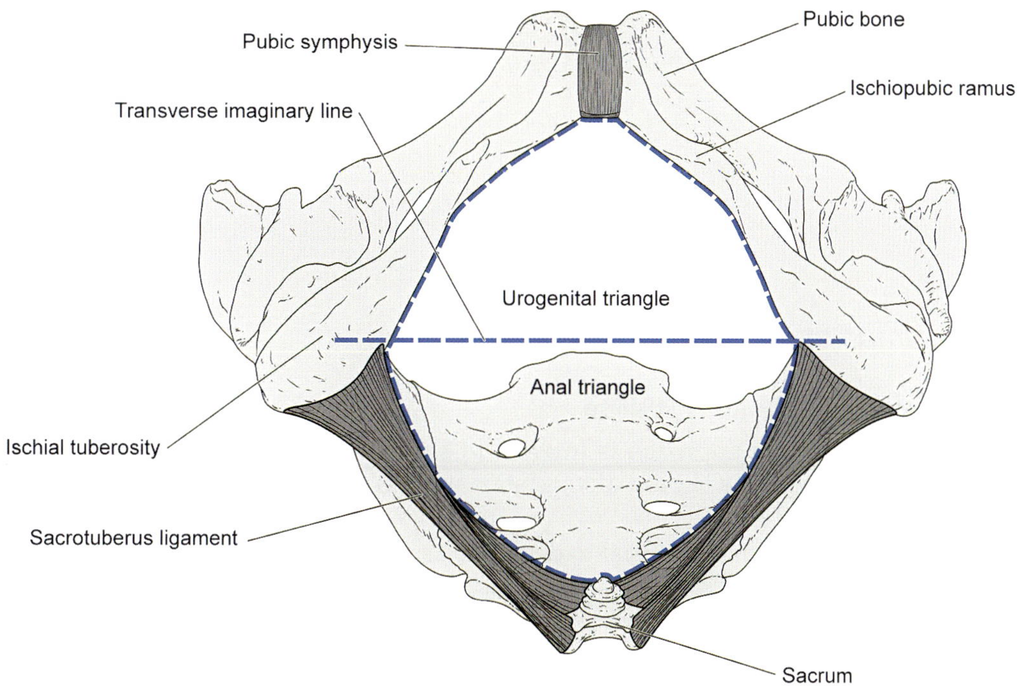

Fig. 4.4: Boundaries of perineum

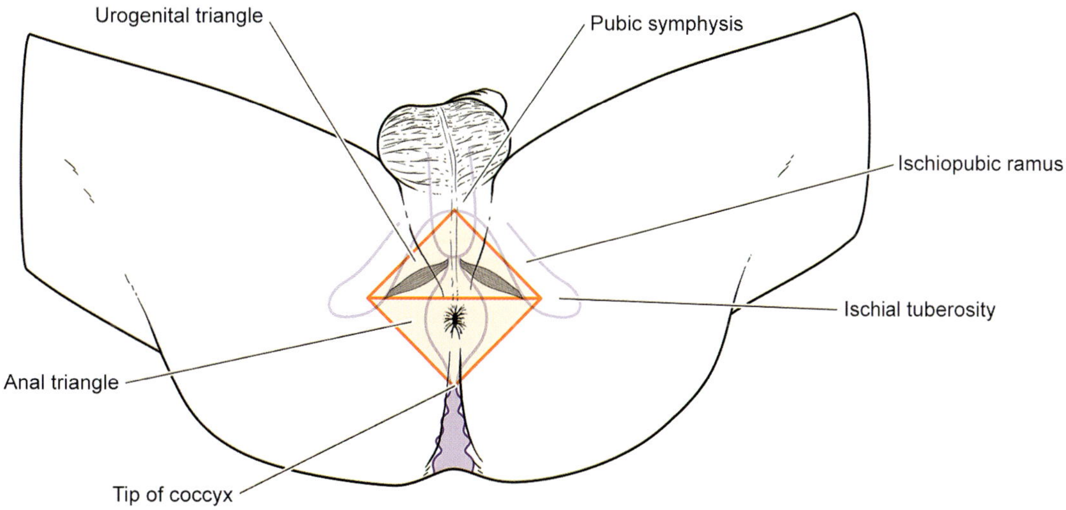

Fig. 4.5: Urogenital and anal triangle

Viewing the Perineum in the Lithotomy Position

While viewing the perineum, the approach is inferior to superior. Whatever is visible first is superficial; anything present above is deep. One should always start with the boundaries of the pelvis to have a better understanding, as shown in Fig. 4.4.

The layers and the contents, from superficial to deep, are as follows:

1. Skin
2. Superficial fatty layer
3. Colles' fascia (continuation of Scarpa's fascia)
4. Superficial perineal pouch
5. Perineal membrane
6. Deep perineal pouch
7. Superior layer of the urogenital diaphragm
8. Pelvic floor muscles
9. Pelvic viscera

The female and male perineum in lithotomy position is shown in Figs 4.6 and 4.7.

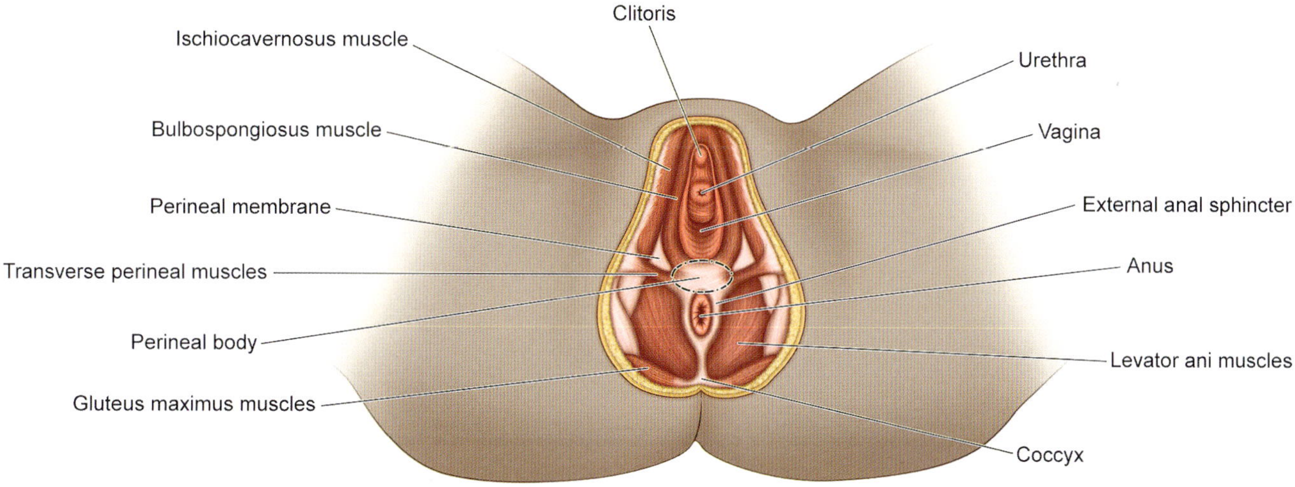

Fig. 4.6: Female perineum

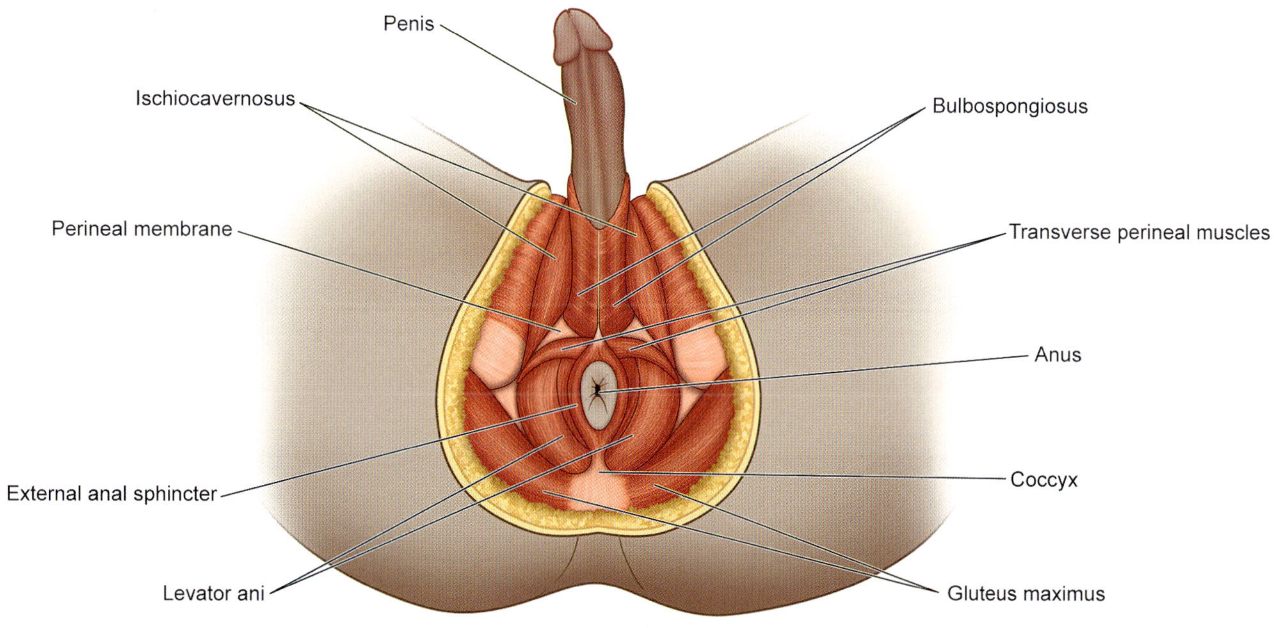

Fig. 4.7: Male perineum

Triangles of Perineum

Urogenital Diaphragm

There are two layers:

- The superior layer
- The inferior layer (also known as the perineal membrane—Fig. 4.8).

Perineal Pouches (Perineal spaces)

Two perineal spaces are critical for determining the extent of the fistula in the anterior region. These spaces are

- Deep perineal space (also known as deep perineal pouch)
- Superficial perineal space (also known as superficial perineal pouch)

The superior layer of the urogenital diaphragm continues with the inferior layer of the urogenital diaphragm (perineal membrane) to form the deep perineal space. The perineal membrane continues with the Colles' fascia (continuation of Scarpa's fascia) to form the superficial perineal pouch (Figure 4.9). As the anterior abdominal wall is deprived of deep fascia, the superficial fascia continues with the deep fascia of the thigh (fascia lata), which forms a pathway for the infection to spread to the medial aspect of the thigh.

Deep Perineal Space

The deep perineal space lies between the superior and inferior layers of the diaphragm.

Boundaries

Roof: Superior layer of urogenital diaphragm

Floor: Inferior layer of urogenital diaphragm (perineal membrane)

Anterior: Transperineal ligament (formed by the fusion of two layers of urogenital diaphragm)

Posterior: Fusion of superior and inferior layers of urogenital diaphragm (Fig. 4.9)

Lateral: Ischiopubic ramus

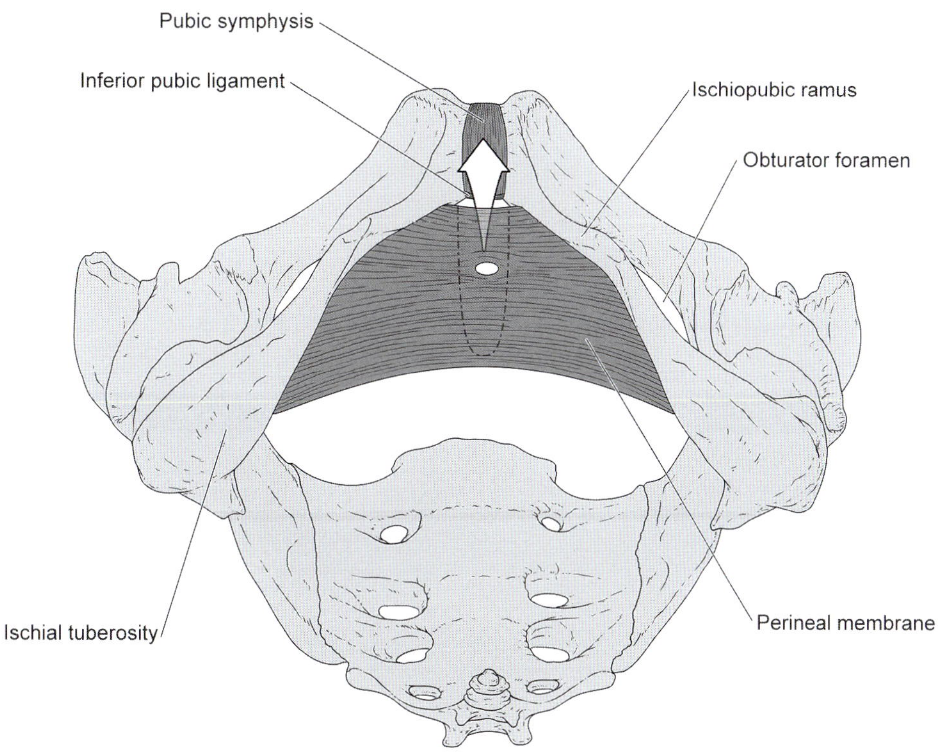

Fig. 4.8: Inferior layer of the urogenital diaphragm (perineal membrane)

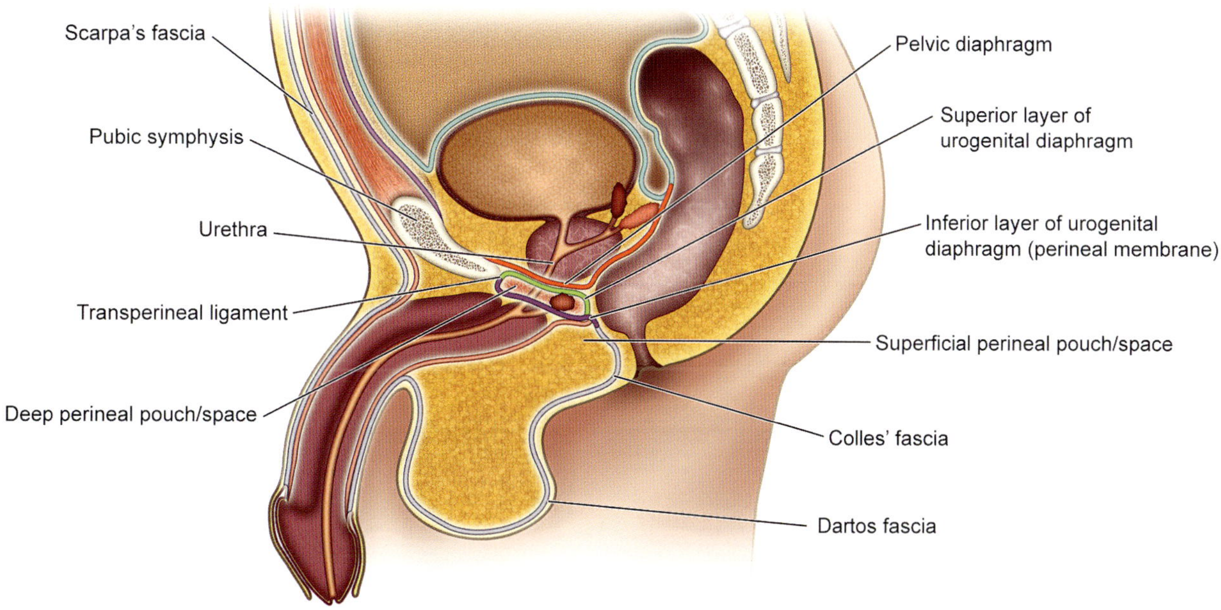

Fig. 4.9: Sagittal section showing fascia and boundaries of the superficial and deep perineal pouch

Contents

Contents of deep perineal pouch in males and females are shown in Table 4.1.

TABLE 4.1: CONTENTS OF DEEP PERINEAL POUCH

Males	*Females*
Membranous urethra (Fig. 4.10A)	Proximal part of the urethra (Fig. 4.10B)
External urethral sphincter	Urtheral and vaginal sphincter
Bulbourethral gland	Compressor urethrae
Deep transverse perineal muscle	Deep transverse perineal muscle
Dorsal nerve of the penis	Dorsal nerve of the clitoris

Clinical Significance of Deep Perineal Space

- Contains bulbourethral glands in males; however, the ducts open in the superficial perineal space.
- The deep transverse perineal muscle plays a role in stabilizing the perineum.

Superficial Perineal Space

This pouch lies between the perineal membrane and the Colles' fascia.

Boundaries

Roof: Perineal membrane

Floor: Colles' fascia

Anterior: Deficient (no boundary as Colles' fascia continues as Scarpa's fascia)

Posterior: Fusion between the layers of Colles' fascia and the perineal membrane (Fig. 4.9)

Lateral: Ischiopubic ramus

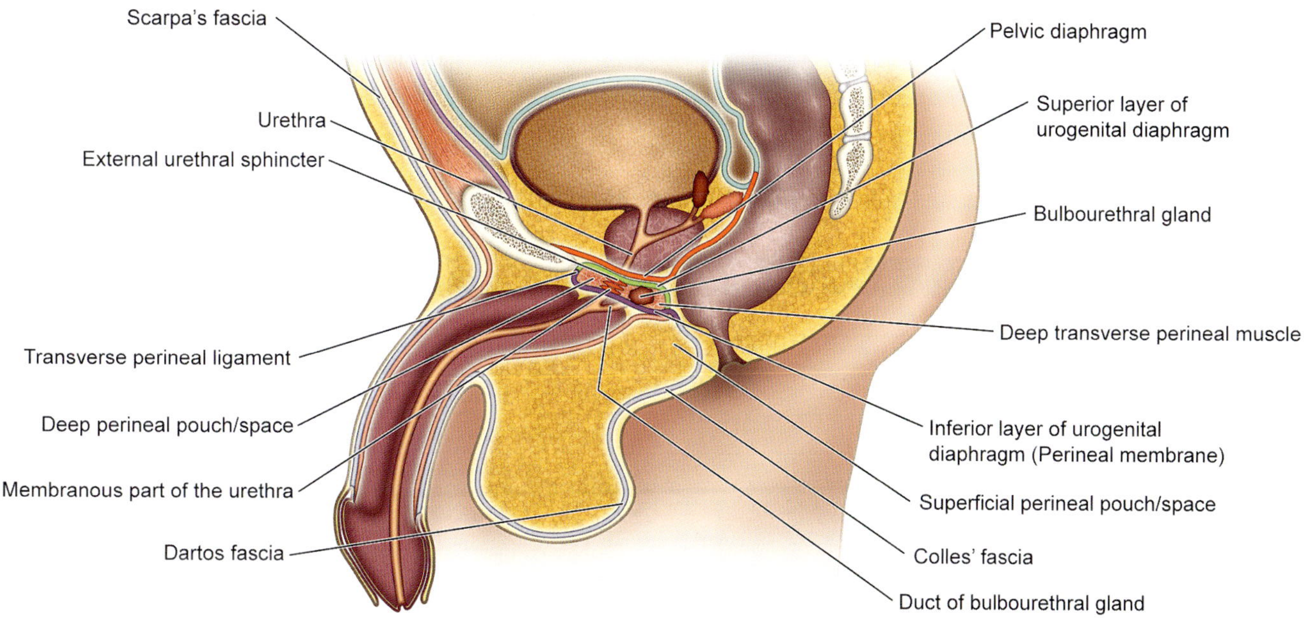

Fig. 4.10A: Sagittal section of the perineum showing the contents of superficial and deep perineal space in males

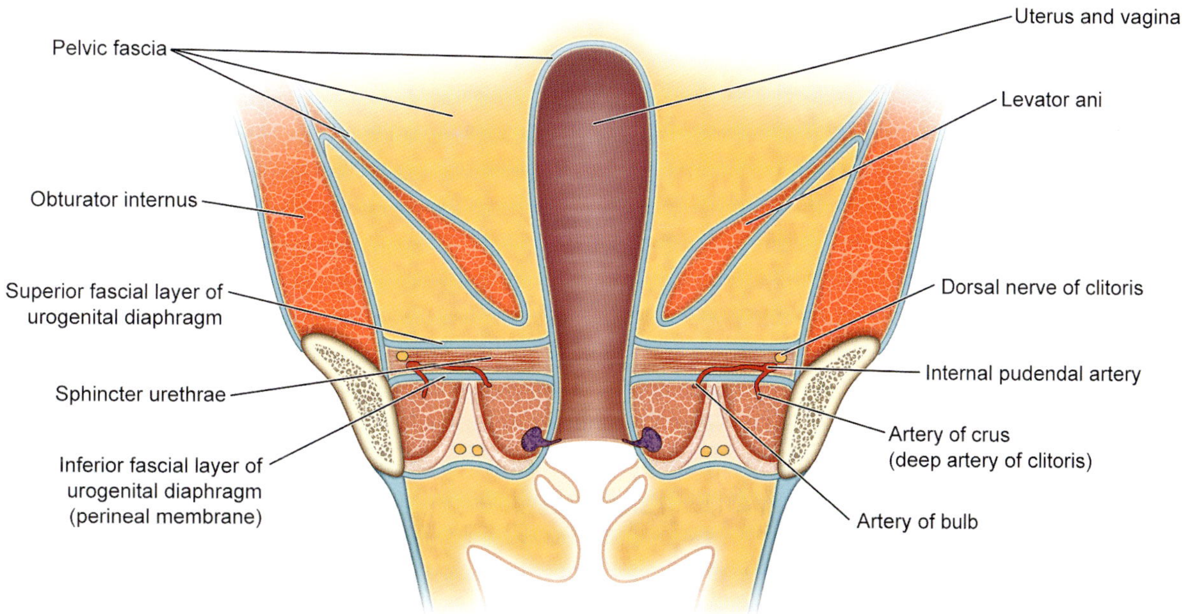

Fig. 4.10B: Coronal section of perineum showing contents of the deep perineal space in females

Superficial Perineal Space

Contents of superficial perineal space in males and females are shown in Table 4.2.

TABLE 4.2: CONTENTS OF SUPERFICIAL PERINEAL SPACE

Males (Fig. 4.11A)	*Females* (Fig. 4.11B)
• Bulbospongiosus	• Bulbospongiosus
• Crus and ischiocavernosus	• Ischiocavernosus
• Anal sphincter	• Anal sphincter
• Superficial transverse perineal muscle	• Superficial transverse perineal muscle
• Levator ani muscles	• Levator ani muscles
• Obturator internus	• Obturator internus
• Perineal body	• Perineal body
• The duct of the bulbourethral gland opens in the bulbous part of the spongy urethra.	• Bartholin's glands (in females)
• Internal pudendal vessels	• Internal pudendal vessels
-	• Vaginal orifice
-	• External urethral orifice
• Posterior scrotal nerve and vessels	• Posterior labial nerve and vessels

Surgical Importance of Superficial Perineal Pouch

- Superficial transverse perineal muscle is important for perineal support and reconstruction during perineal repair.
- Anterior spread of fistulas takes place into the superficial perineal space through Colles' fascia. The spread occurs between the superficial and deep transverse perineal muscles.

Surgical Importance of the Pouches in Relation to Urethral Injury

- Injury to the membranous part of the urethra will cause urine accumulation in the deep perineal pouch.
- Injury to the spongy part of the urethra will cause extravasation of urine into the superficial pouch, scrotum, and lower anterior abdominal wall.

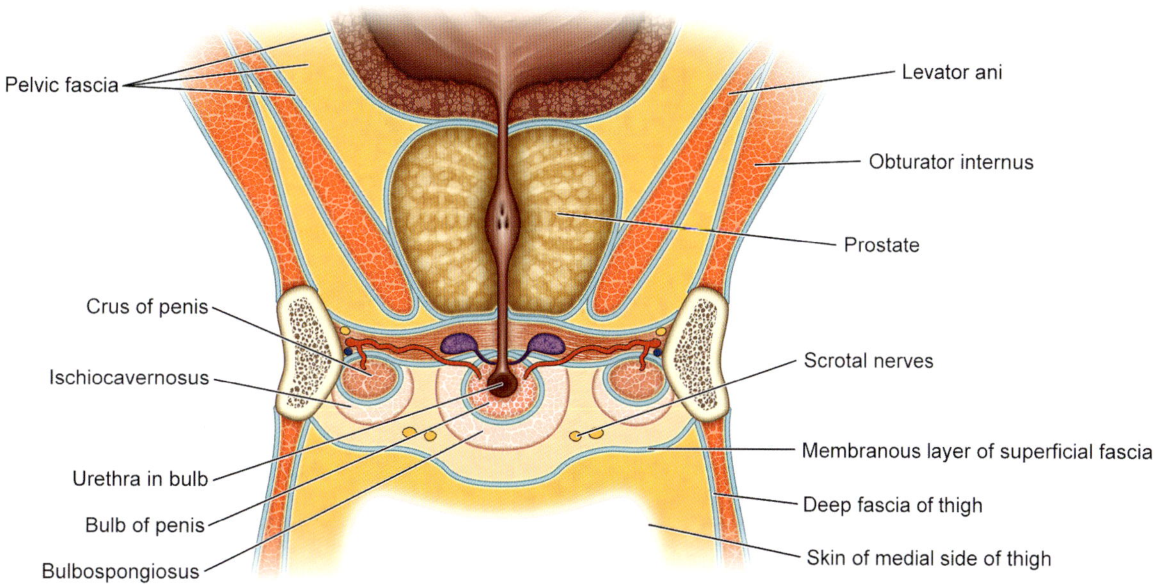

Fig. 4.11A: Contents of the superficial perineal pouch in males

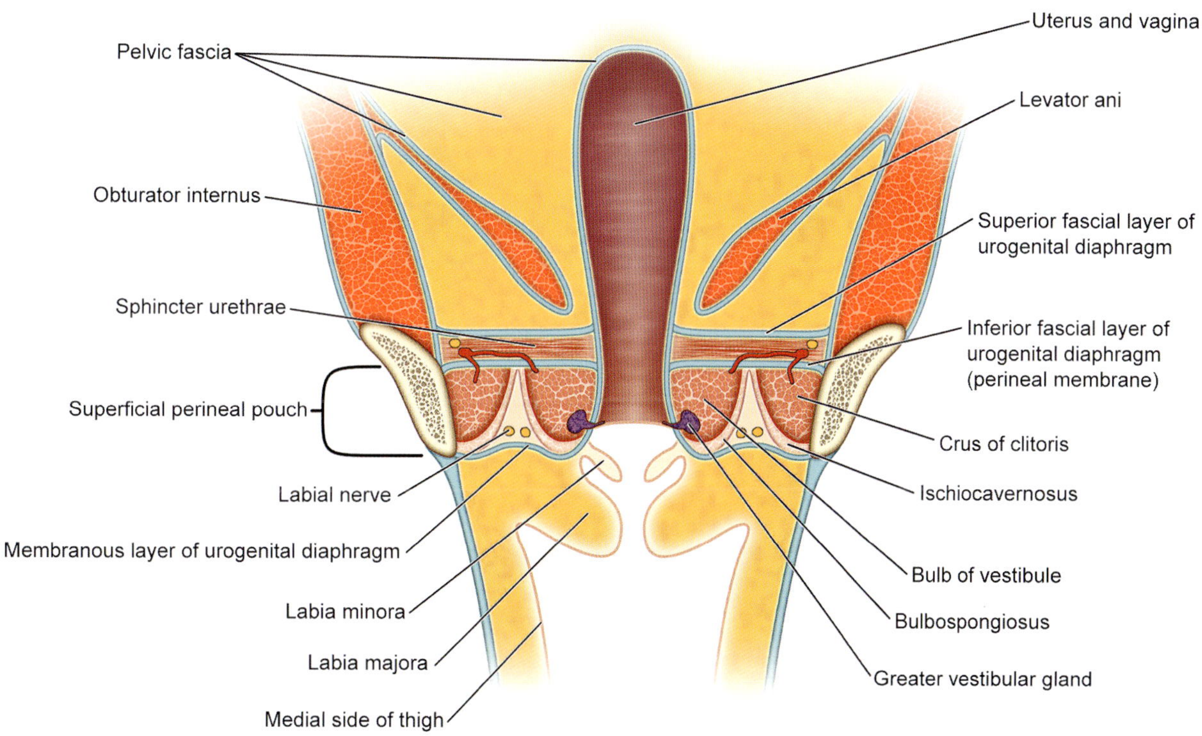

Fig. 4.11B: Contents of the superficial perineal space in females

Fascias and their Correlation with the Anterior Fistulas

- The Colles' fascia forms the floor of the superficial perineal space, continuous as the Dartos fascia and then as the Scarpa's fascia of the lower abdominal wall. Since the superficial perineal pouch has no anterior boundary, the anterior fistulas may extend through this space and present as an external opening at the penoscrotal junction or the lower abdominal wall.
- The lateral extension of the anterior tracts may give rise to an external opening in the medial aspect of the thigh where the Scarpa's fascia merges with the fascia lata in the upper thigh (Fig. 4.12A and B)

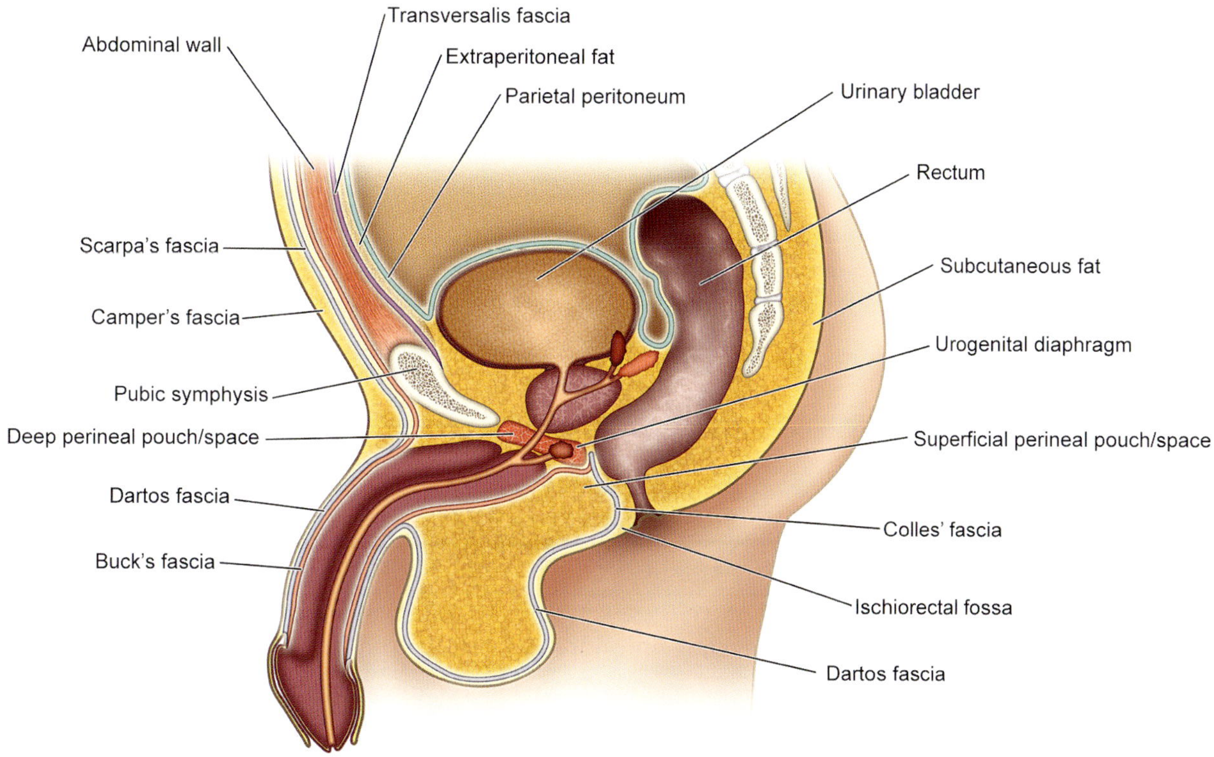

Fig. 4.12A: Fascias and their correlations in the perineum

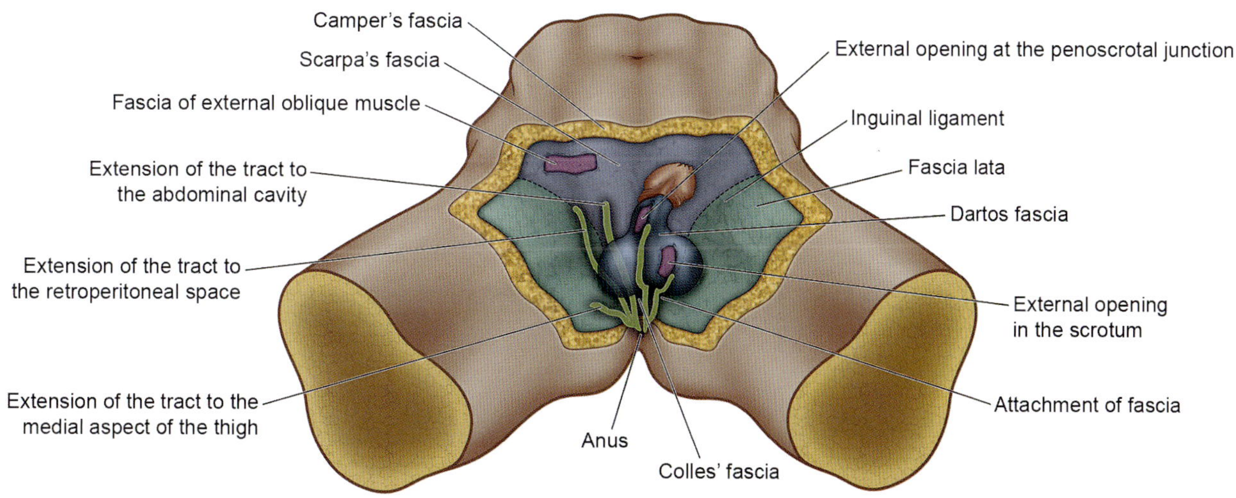

Fig. 4.12B: Fascias and their correlations in the perineum showing extensions of fistula tracts

A WORD ABOUT BULBOURETHRAL AND BARTHOLIN GLAND

Bulbourethral Gland

Location

- In the deep perineal pouch in males.
- Posterior and lateral to the membranous portion of the urethra at the base of the penis (Fig. 4.13).

Ducts

The ducts pierce the perineal membrane to open into the bulbous urethra in the superficial perineal pouch.

> **Surgical Significance**
>
> A bulbourethral abscess can appear as a swelling in the scrotum.

How to Differentiate Bulbourethral Abscess and Anterior Anal Fistula

An infection of the bulbourethral gland can be misinterpreted as an anterior anal fistula. The fistula tract is palpable as a thick fibrous cord with an internal and an external opening. The patient can be subjected to MRI to confirm the diagnosis.

Bartholin Gland

Location

- In the superficial perineal pouch in females.
- In the vulvar vestibule (at either side of the labia majora).

> **Surgical Significance**
>
> Sometimes the openings of these glands become obstructed, leading to the formation of Bartholin's cyst or abscess.

How to Differentiate Bartholin Cyst and the Anterior Anal Fistula

An infection of the Bartholin gland can be misinterpreted as an external opening of an anal fistula. Bartholin cyst or abscess presents as a painful swelling in the posterolateral wall near the labia. The most typical site of cyst formation is in the lower one-third of the vagina. In contrast, the fistulous opening in the perianal region communicates with the anal canal. The fistula tract is palpable as a thick fibrous cord with an internal and an external opening. Another diagnostic tool is MRI (Fig. 4.14).

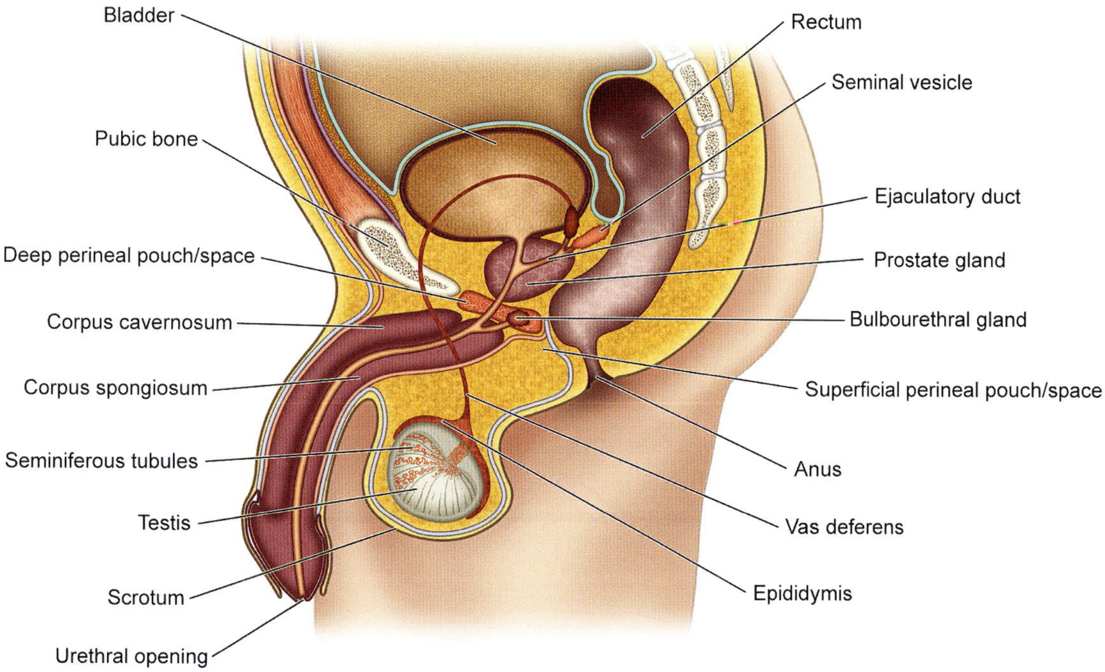

Fig. 4.13: Bulbourethral gland

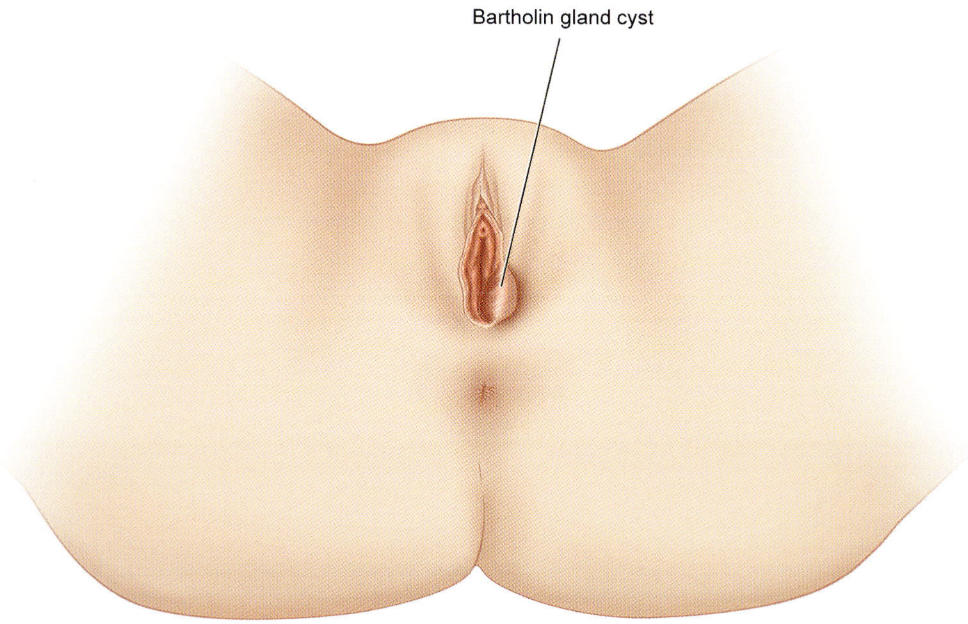

Fig. 4.14: Bartholin gland cyst

Important Surgical Considerations

Perineal Body

The fusion of the fibres of the following muscles forms the perineal body:

- Superficial part of the external anal sphincter
- Superficial and deep transverse perineal muscles
- Levator ani
- Bulbospongiosus
- Compressor urethra muscle
- Internal anal sphincter muscle attached posteriorly to the perineal body
- External urethral muscle
- Retrouretheralis muscle
- Conjoined longitudinal muscle (Fig. 4.15)

Fascial Structures Joining the Perineal Body

- *Anteriorly:* Superficial perineal fascia.
- *Superiorly:* Rectovaginal fascia in females and rectoprostatic septum in males.

Conclusion

Inflammation and infection of cryptoglandular or non-cryptoglandular origin in the anal canal can quickly spread to the perineum. It is, therefore, imperative to know the anatomy of this region to understand the spread of anorectal abscesses and fistulas.

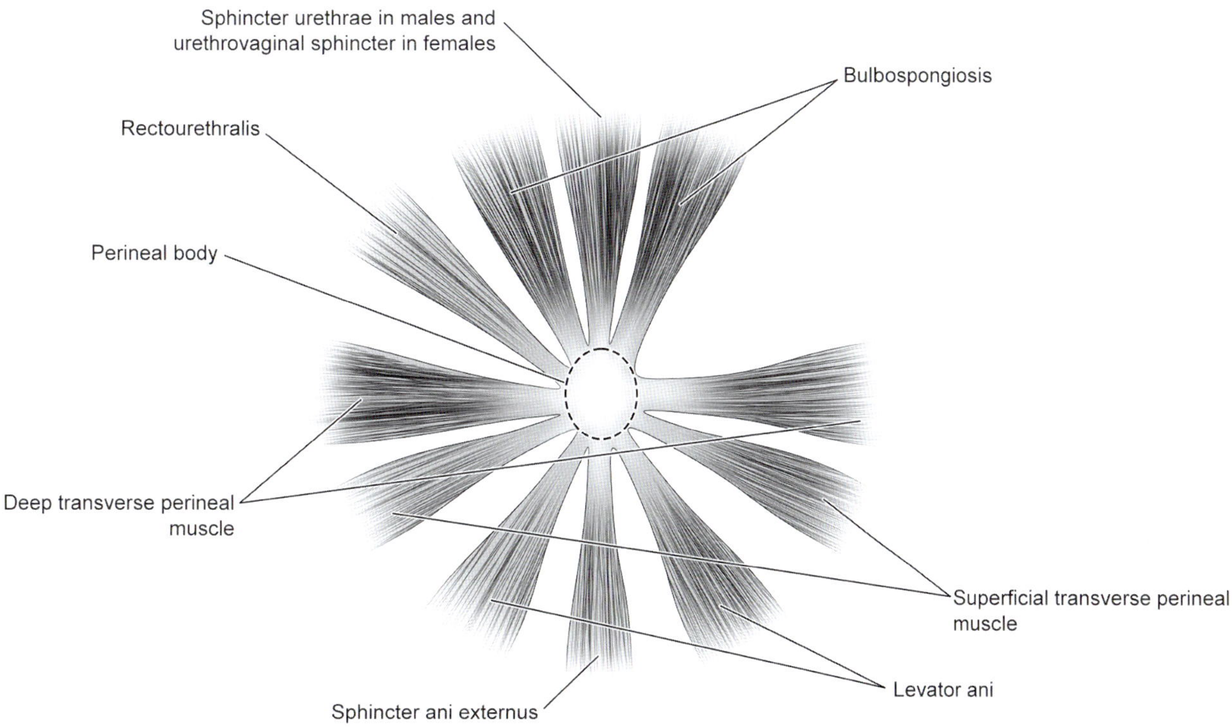

Fig. 4.15: Diagram showing the muscle insertion in the perineal body

Further Reading

- Anatomy, Abdomen, and Pelvis: Superficial Perineal Space Michael W. Fahmy; Tanisha Sanganeria; Sunil Munakomi.
- Anatomy, Abdomen and Pelvis, Perineal Body.Marco A. Siccardi; Bruno Bordoni.
- Functional anatomy of female perineum https://www.intechopen.com/online-first/83986.
- Functional Anatomy of Female Perineum October 2022
- Oh C, Kark AE. Anatomy of the perineal body. Dis Colon Rectum 16, 444–454 (1973). https://doi.org/10.1007/BF02588867
- Perineum an overview https://www.sciencedirect.com/topics/medicine-and-dentistry/perineum
- The perineum https://teachmeanatomy.info/pelvis/areas/perineum/

CHAPTER 5

Pathophysiology of Anal Abscess

Abscesses and anal fistulas are anorectal suppurative disorders representing two phases of the same disease. Anal abscess symbolises the "acute phase," while the fistula represents the "chronic phase". They frequently coexist. Approximately 95% of abscesses and fistulas are cryptoglandular, while the remaining are due to conditions like Crohn's disease, inflammatory bowel disease and tuberculosis.

The anal glands within the anal crypts play a crucial role in forming anorectal abscesses; therefore, it is imperative to have a basic understanding of the anatomy of the anal glands.

Anatomy of Anal Glands

- The anal glands are around 6–8 in number and are primarily located posteriorly.
- About 80% of the glands are in the submucosa, and 8% are in the intersphincteric space (Fig. 5.1).
- The ducts of the anal glands open at the dentate line.
- These glands may be tubular or branched.
- Each gland produces 4–16 secondary and tertiary ramifications. Most of these branches run caudally (Fig. 5.2).
- The ramifications create pathways for the infection to spread. The greater the number of channels, the greater the possibility of the spread of infection (Fig. 5.2).
- Anal glands are referred to as "anal tonsils" because of the presence of lymphoid follicles.

Location of Anal Glands (Table 5.1)

TABLE 5.1: PERCENT PENETRATION OF ANAL GLANDS

Penetration of the gland	*Percentage*
Submucosal	80
Intersphincteric	8
Conjoined longitudinal muscle	7–8
External anal sphincter	1

Length of the Duct

1–2 mm. In some cases, it may be 4 mm.

Direction of Anal Glands

- Usually caudal
- Rarely lateral or cephalad

Lining of Anal Glands

- Stratified columnar epithelium with mucus secreting cells

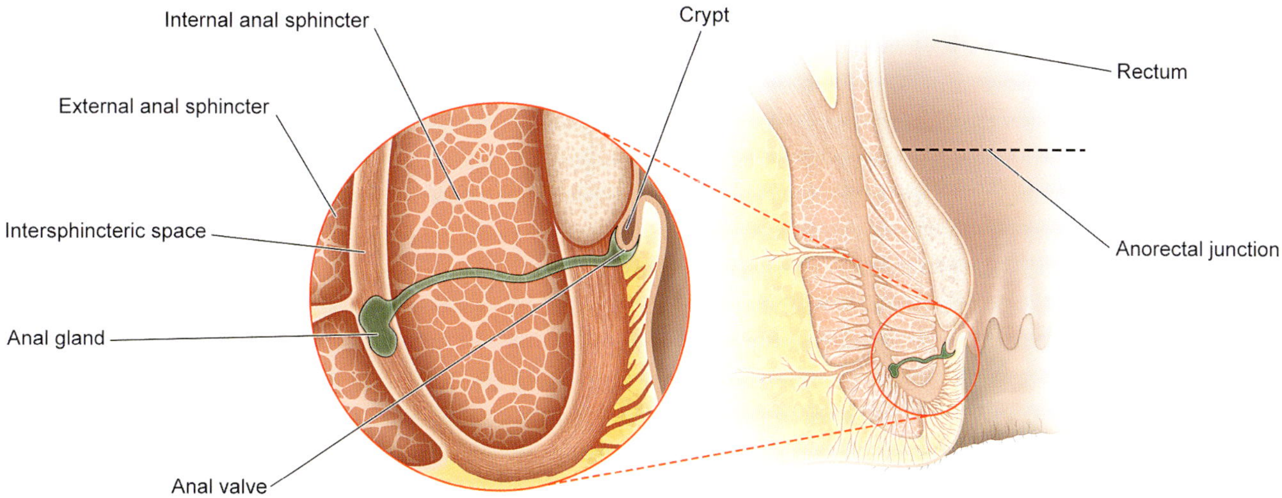

Fig. 5.1: Diagrammatic representation of the anal gland opening in the intersphincteric space

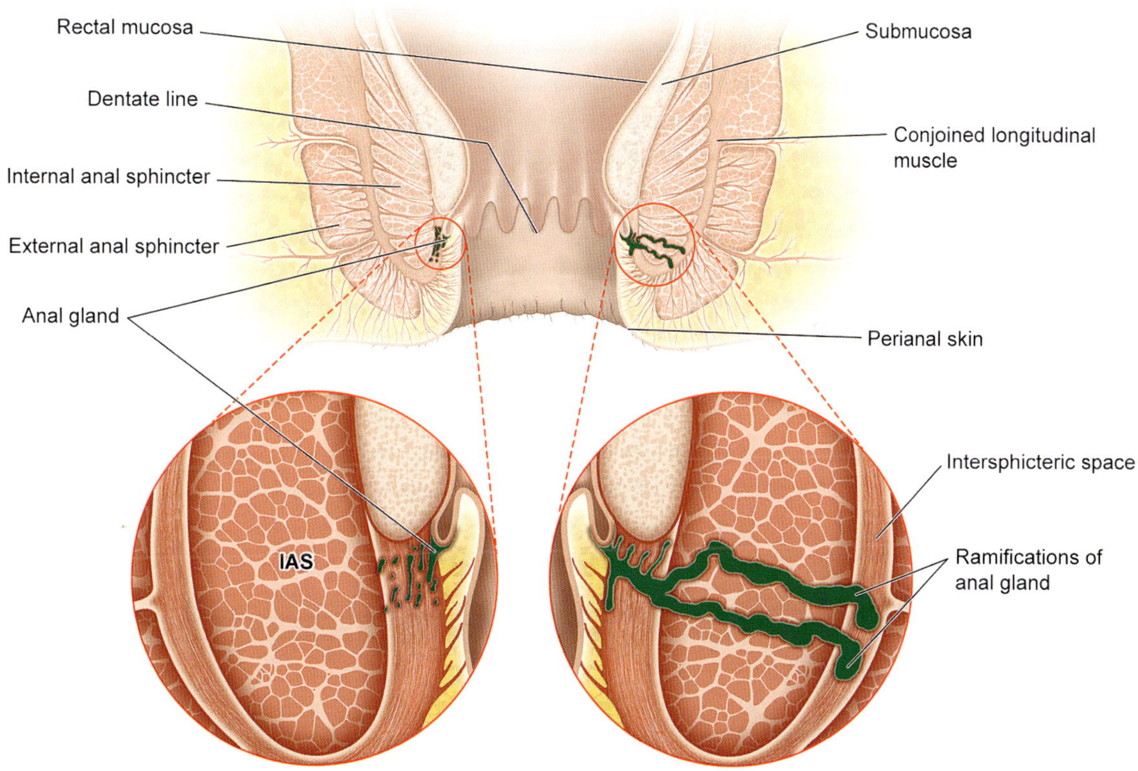

Fig. 5.2: Diagrammatic representation of the anal glands in submucosal and intersphincteric space

Pathophysiology of Abscess and Fistula Formation

Phase 1: Abscess and fistula formation starts with obstruction (fecal impaction) in the anal gland duct (Fig. 5.3).

Phase 2: This may result in stasis and cyst formation, primarily if the affected gland produces mucus. The cyst is usually 5 mm in diameter (Fig. 5.3).

Phase 3: The cyst may become infected, and the infected material, including bacteria, cellular debris, and inflammatory cells, accumulates within the lumen, leading to enlargement and subsequent rupture of the epithelial wall. This may lead to abscess and subsequent fistula formation (Fig. 5.4). The infected cyst acts as a nidus of infection.

Most anal ducts have their outlet posteriorly in the anal canal. Sometimes multiple ducts may open in a single anal crypt.

Fate of Anal Glands

The obstruction of the anal gland duct can lead to

- Stasis
- Infection
- Abscess or fistula formation

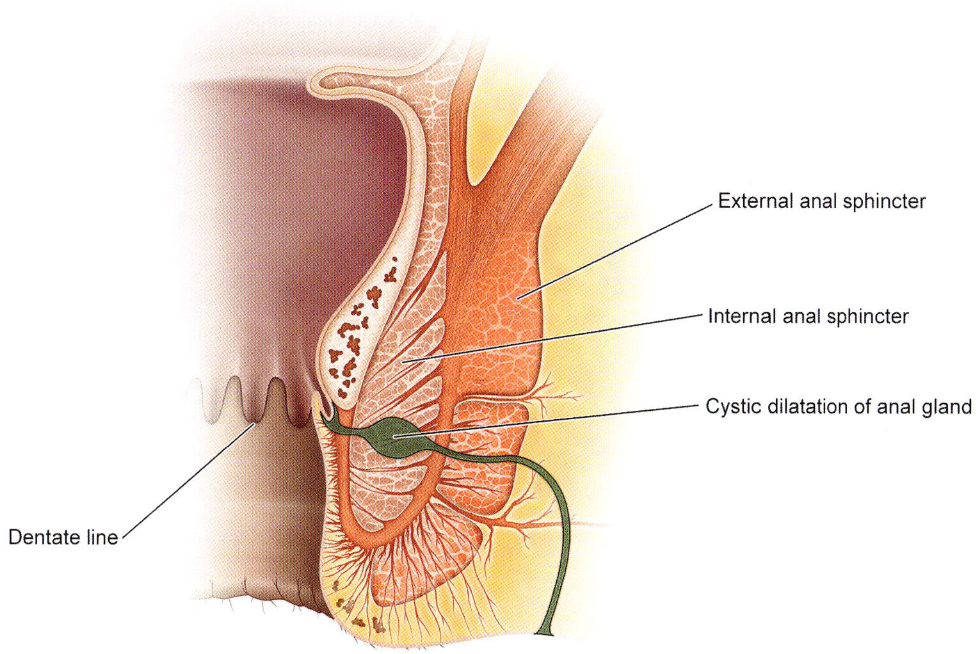

Fig. 5.3: Intersphincteric dilatation of the anal duct (cyst formation)

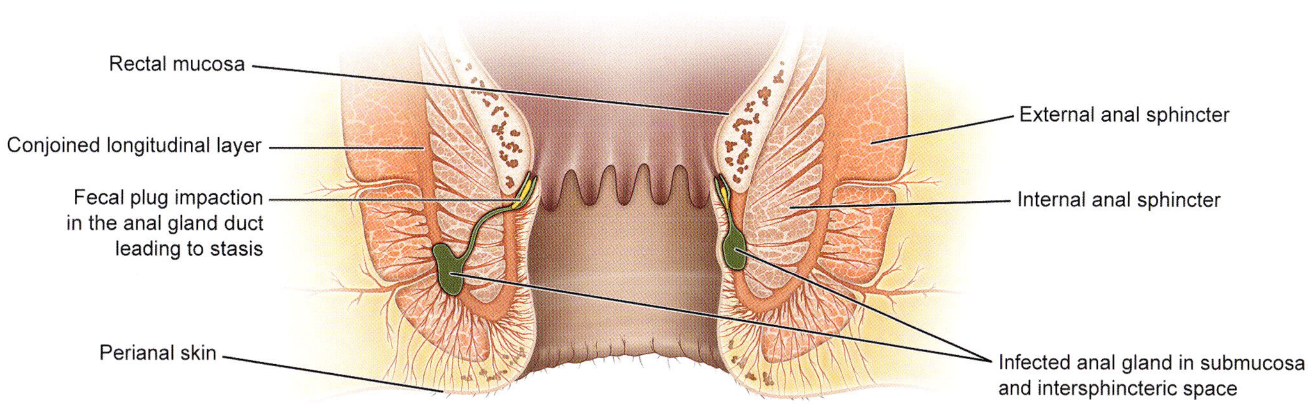

Fig. 5.4: Diagram illustrating the mode of abscess formation from the anal glands

Pathways of Spread of an Abscess

The infection spreads through the following pathways:

- Superficial or submucosal pathways
- Between the internal and external sphincters
- Across the sphincters (trans-sphincteric or suprasphincteric)
- Anteriorly after crossing the transverse perineal muscles
- Posteriorly towards the sacrotuberous ligament and gluteus maximus

Types of Abscesses

Depending on the path followed, different types of abscesses and fistulas are formed (Fig. 5.5). These are as follows:

- Submucosal
- Intersphincteric
- Perianal
- Ischiorectal
- Supralevator

Formation of Different Types of Abscesses

Submucosal Abscess

- When the submucosal gland becomes infected, it forms a submucosal abscess. It discharges spontaneously into the anal canal (Fig. 5.6).

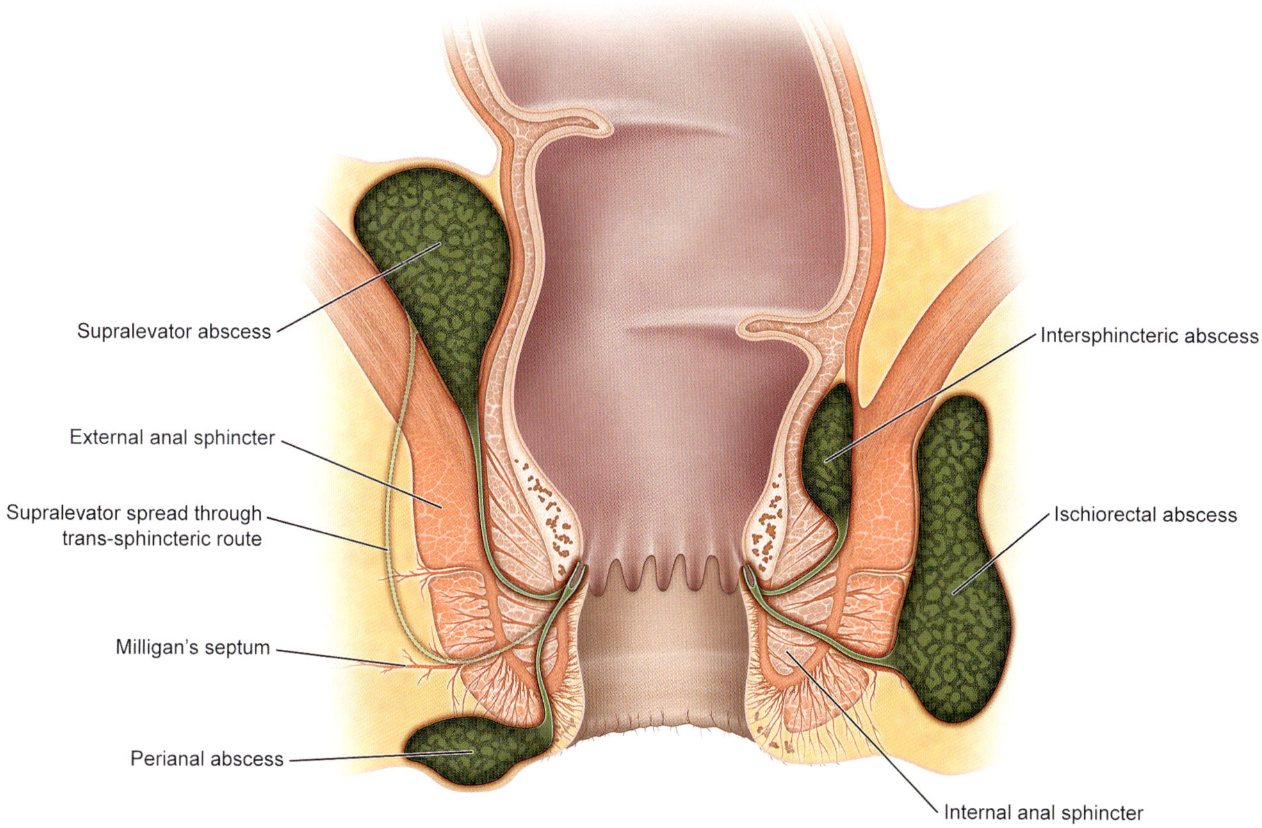

Fig. 5.5: Different types of abscesses

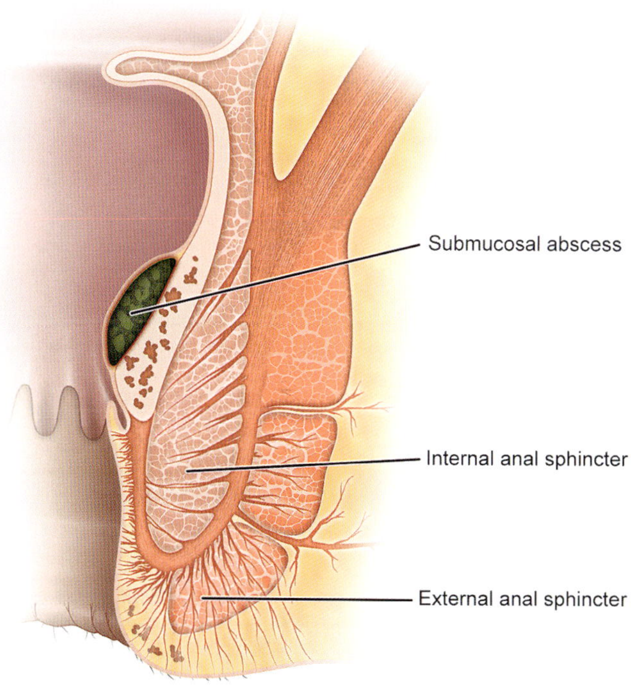

Fig. 5.6: Submucosal abscess

Intersphincteric Abscess

An intersphincteric abscess is formed in the intersphincteric space between the internal and the external anal sphincters (Fig. 5.7). Depending on the direction of ramifications, the abscess may spread caudally to discharge spontaneously into the perianal space, forming an intersphincteric abscess or fistula. An upward extension can lead to the formation of a suprasphincteric abscess.

Perianal Abscess

A perianal abscess forms when the intersphincteric abscess extends downward toward the perianal space (Fig. 5.8).

Ischiorectal Abscess

When the infection spreads through the external anal sphincter, it forms an ischiorectal abscess (Fig. 5.9).

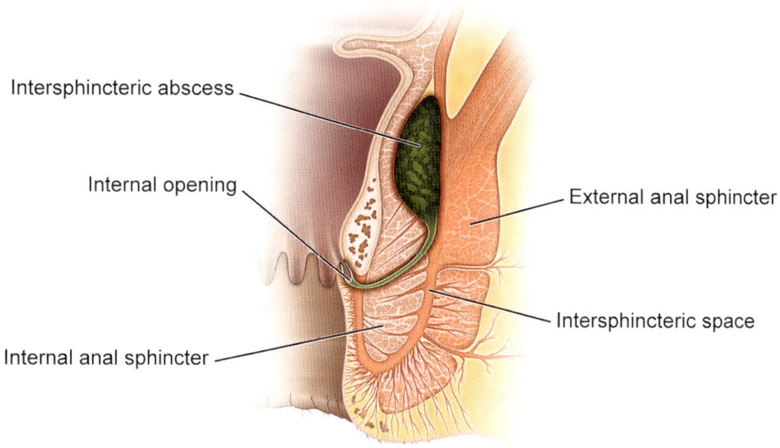

Fig. 5.7: Intersphincteric abscess

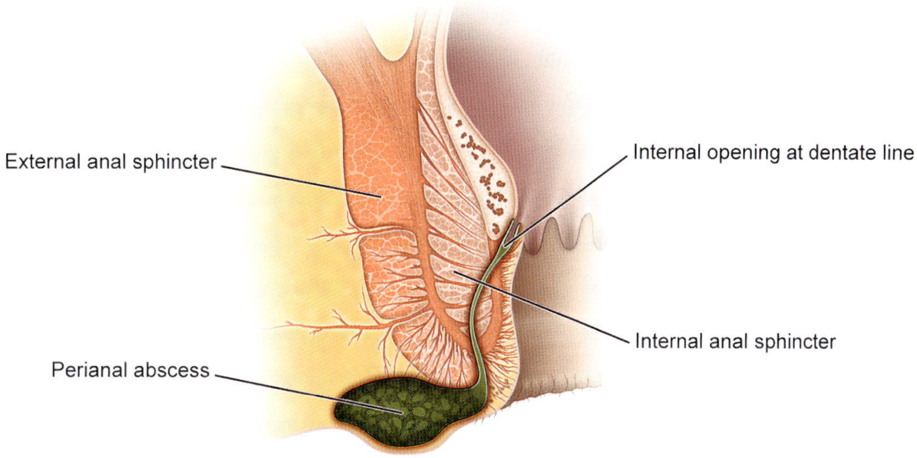

Fig. 5.8: Perianal abscess with communicating low intersphincteric fistula

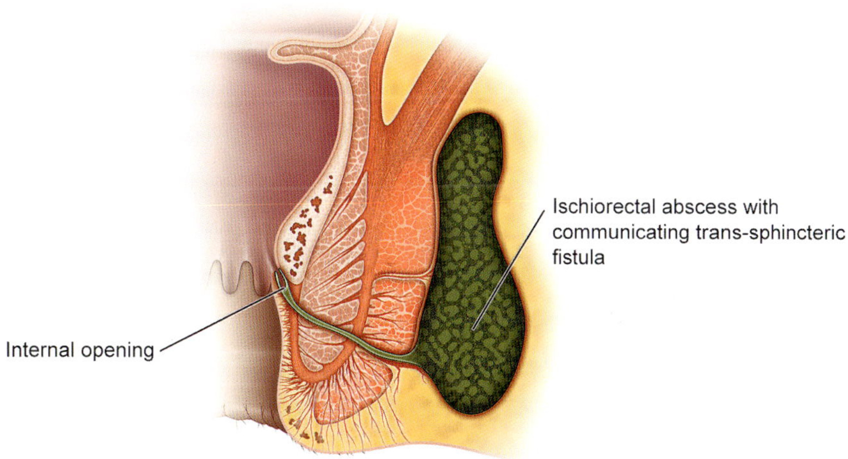

Fig. 5.9: Ischiorectal abscess communicating with the anal canal

Supralevator Abscess

- A cephalad spread of an intersphincteric abscess towards the levators can lead to a supralevator abscess (Fig. 5.10A).
- A downward extension from the pelvic infection can also lead to a supralevator abscess (Fig. 5.10B).
- An ischiorectal abscess can extend through the ischiorectal septum into the infralevator space. Rarely, the infralevator abscess can pierce the fascia lunata and the infralevator fascia to extend into the supralevator space (Fig. 5.10C).

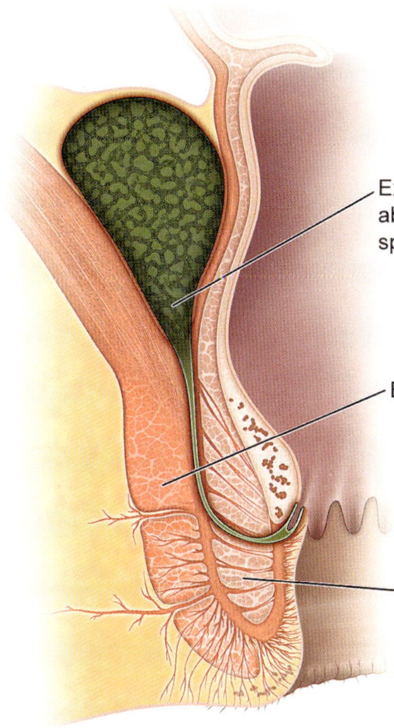

Fig. 5.10A: Cephalad spread of an intersphincteric abscess forming supralevator abscess

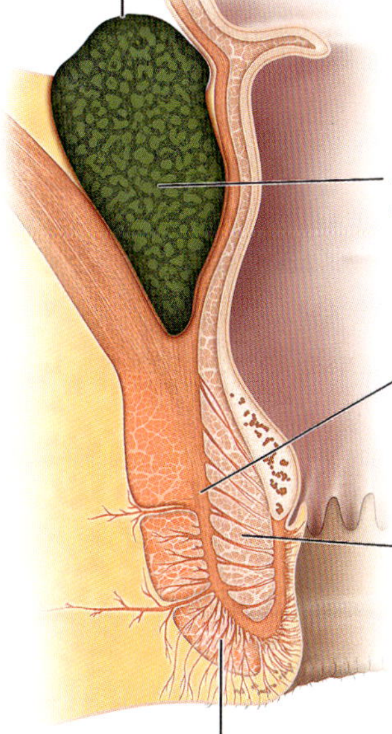

Fig. 5.10B: Supralevator abscess formed as a result of downward extension from the pelvis

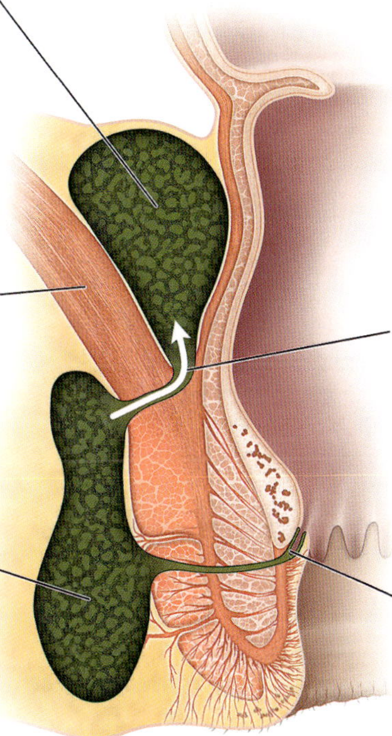

Fig. 5.10C: Upward extension from ischiorectal abscess through the levators forming supralevator abscess

Surgical Significance of Anal Glands

One should remember that once the infection sets in, the anal gland gets dissolved and forms an abscess which acts as a nidus. Surgical management of an anorectal abscess involves removing the nidus and achieving adequate drainage. During the procedure, the surgeon must identify all the extensions to ensure complete drainage of the abscess cavity. Failure to adequately drain the abscess can result in persistent infection, incomplete resolution, and an increased risk of developing recurrent abscesses or fistulas.

Two techniques are used to tackle the primary source of infection:

- Park's technique advocates the complete removal of the infected gland, internal opening, and opening of the deep intersphincter space (Figs 5.11 and 5.12).
- Eisenhammer recommends laying open the tract from external to the internal opening and curetting the nidus of infection. According to him the anal gland gets dissolved, once the infection sets in (Fig. 5.13).

Correlation with Tuberculosis, Crohn's Disease, Ulcerative Colitis, and Carcinoma Rectum

- The anal glands are surrounded by lymphatic tissue, which explains the association of anal abscesses with tuberculosis and Crohn's disease.
- Ian MacColl reported that anal glands are not involved in ulcerative colitis. It is the mucosa and submucosa that showed inflammatory changes in ulcerative colitis.
- The anal glands may rarely give rise to adenocarcinoma.

Conclusion

The surgical importance of anal glands is attributed to their role in the pathogenesis of anorectal abscesses and fistulas. Anorectal abscesses are common surgical presentations resulting from obstruction or infection of the anal glands. A surgeon must understand the anatomy and pathophysiology of these glands to ensure proper identification of the type of abscesses and the pathways of spread. Any nidus of infection left behind during surgical management will lead to a chronic stage where the patient may develop recurrent abscesses or fistula formation.

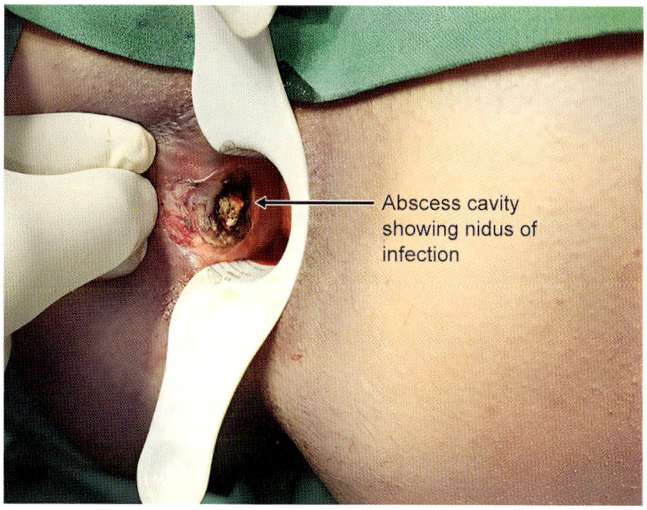

Fig. 5.11: Abscess cavity showing nidus of infection

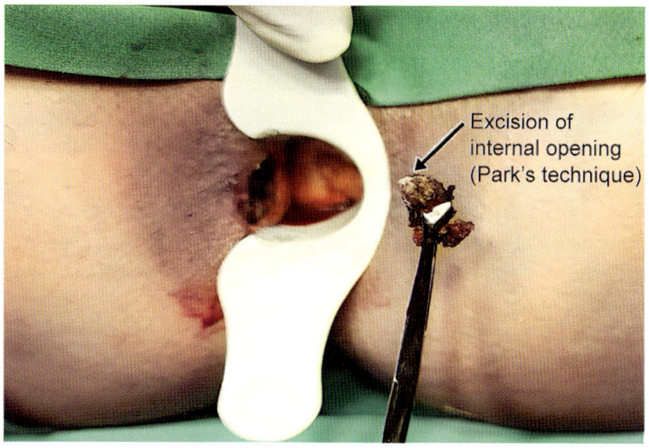

Fig. 5.12: Park's technique—complete removal of the gland and the internal opening

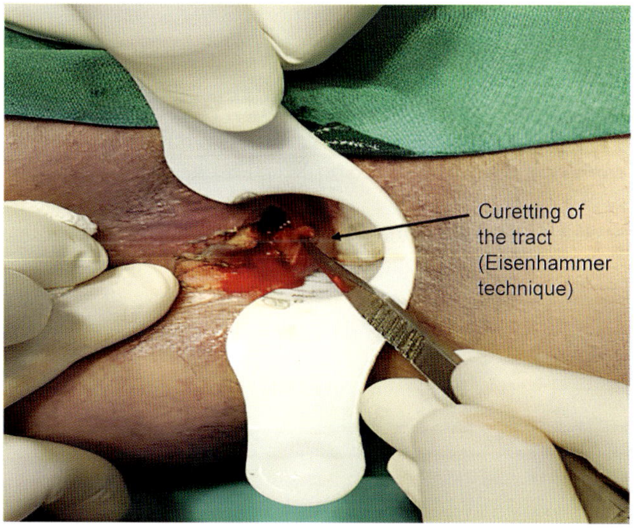

Fig. 5.13: Eisenhammer technique—laying open of the tract followed by curetting

Further Reading

- Adamo K, Sandblom G, Brännström F, Strigård K. Prevalence and recurrence rate of perianal abscess--a population-based study, Sweden 1997-2009. Int J Colorectal Dis. 2016 Mar;31(3):669–73. doi 10.1007/s00384-015-2500-7. Epub 2016 Jan 14. PMID: 26768004.
- Aspects of fistula-in-ano Pdf by PJ Lunnis.
- Brook I. The role of anaerobic bacteria in cutaneous and soft tissue abscesses and infected cysts. Anaerobe. 2007 Oct-Dec;13(5-6):171–7. [PubMed]
- Duhamel J. Anal fistulae in childhood. Am J Proctol. 1975 Dec;26(6):40–3. PMID: 1211441.
- Eglitis JA, & Eglitis, I. (1961). The glands of the anal canal in man.[Google Scholar].
- EISENHAMMER S. The internal anal sphincter; its surgical importance. S Afr Med J. 1953 Mar 28;27(13):266–70. PMID: 13076663.
- EISENHAMMER S. The internal anal sphincter and the anorectal abscess. Surg Gynecol Obstet. 1956 Oct;103(4):501–6. PMID: 13360660.
- Goligher JC, Ellis M, Pissidis AG. A critique of anal glandular infection in the etiology and treatment of idiopathic anorectal abscesses and fistulas. Br J Surg. 1967 Dec;54(12):977–83. doi: 10.1002/bjs.1800541202. PMID: 6066322.
- Hanley PH. Reflections on anorectal abscess fistula: 1984. Dis Colon Rectum. 1985 Jul;28(7):528–33. doi 10.1007/BF02554105. PMID: 3893948.[PubMed]
- Herand Abcarian Relationship of Abscess and Fistula. Anal Fistula: Principles and Management, DOI 10. 1007/978-1-4614-9014-2-3
- Kinugasa Y, Arakawa T, Abe H, Abe S, Cho BH, Murakami G, Sugihara K. Anococcygeal raphe revisited: a histological study using mid-term human fetuses and elderly cadavers. Yonsei Med J. 2012 Jul 1;53(4):849–55. doi: 10.3349/ymj.2012.53.4.849. PMID: 22665356; PMCID: PMC3381476.
- ML Prasad, DR Read, and H. Abcarian, "Supralevator abscess: diagnosis and treatment," Diseases of the Colon and Rectum, vol. 24, no. 6, pp. 456–61, 1981. View at:[Google Scholar]
- Parks AG, Gordon PH, Hardcastle JD. A classification of fistula-in-ano. Br J Surg. 1776 Jan;63(1):1–12. DOI: 10.1002/bjs.1800630102. PMID: 1267867.[PubMed].
- Parks AG, Gordon PH, Hardcastle JD. A classification of fistula-in-ano. Br J Surg. 1976 Jan;63(1):1-12. doi: 10.1002/bjs.1800630102. PMID: 1267867.
- PARKS AG. Pathogenesis and treatment of fistula-in-ano. Br Med J. 1961 Feb 18;1(5224):463–9. Doi: 10.1136/bmj.1.5224.463. PMID: 13732880; PMCID: PMC1953161.
- Ramanujam PS, Prasad ML, Abcarian H, Tan AB. Perianal abscesses and fistulas. A study of 1023 patients. Dis Colon Rectum. 1984 Sep;27(9):593–7. doi 10.1007/BF02553848. PMID: 6468199.[PubMed]
- Sanyal S, Khan F, Ramachandra P. Successful management of a recurrent supralevator abscess: a case report. Case Rep Surg. 2012;2012:871639. Doi: 10.1155/2012/871639. Epub 2012 May 7. PMID: 22649747; PMCID: PMC3357932.
- Seow-Choen F, Ho JM. Histoanatomy of anal glands. Dis Colon Rectum. 1774 Dec;37(12):1215–8. doi 10.1007/BF02257784. PMID: 7775146.[Pubmed]
- Sigmon DF, Emmanuel B, Tuma F. Perianal Abscess. 2021 June 27. In: StatPearls [Internet]. Treasure Island (FL): StatPearls Publishing; 2021 Jan–. PMID: 27083652.[PubMed]
- Turner SV, Singh J. Perirectal Abscess. 2021 Aug 11. In: StatPearls [Internet]. Treasure Island (FL): StatPearls Publishing; 2022 Jan–. PMID: 29939672.[PubMed]
- Ustynoski K, Rosen L, Stasik J, Riether R, Sheets J, Khubchandani IT. Horseshoe abscess fistula. Seton treatment. Dis Colon Rectum. 1990 Jul;33(7):602–5. doi: 10.1007/BF02052216. PMID: 2361430.
- Whiteford MH. Perianal abscess/fistula disease. Clin Colon Rectal Surg. 2007 May;20(2):102–7. doi 10.1055/s-2007-777488. PMID: 20011384; PMCID: PMC2780182
- Whiteford MH. Perianal abscess/fistula disease. Clin Colon Rectal Surg. 2007 May;20(2):102–9. doi: 10.1055/s-2007-977488. PMID: 20011384; PMCID: PMC2780182.[PubMed]

CHAPTER 6

Pathways of Spread of Anorectal Abscesses and Fistulas

Once a surgeon gets familiar with the anatomy of the perineum, and the pathophysiology of anorectal abscesses and fistulas, it becomes easy to understand the pathways of spread.

The anatomy of the anal musculature remains constant. According to Kurihara, the infection spreads through musculature and the fascias, following the path of least resistance.

Eisenhammer stated, "A faulty surgery may lead to disruption of the natural pathways and open new planes for the spread of infection leading to complicated anorectal abscesses and fistulas".

Spread of Infection from the Anal Canal to the Surrounding Tissues

An abscess tends to follow the path of least resistance along specific anatomical pathways. The arrangement of the muscle fibres in the CLM play a crucial role in spreading infection from the anal canal to the surrounding tissues to form an abscess or a fistula. The fibres of CLM pass inward through the internal anal sphincter muscle and outward through the external anal sphincter muscle. This allows the infection to extend directly from the anal canal into the perianal and ischiorectal spaces (Fig. 6.1A and B).

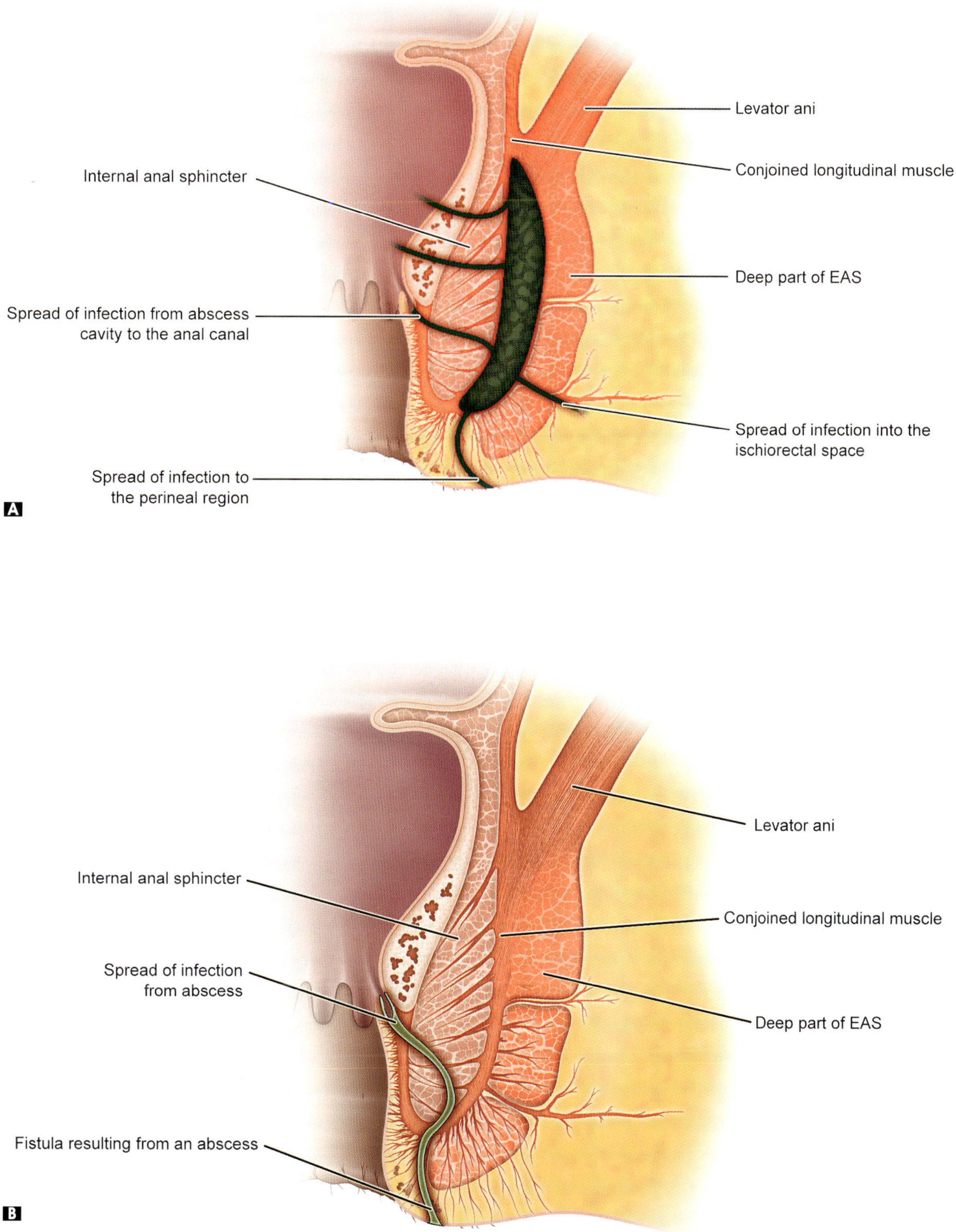

Fig. 6.1: Diagrammatic representation of the spread of infection resulting in fistula formation

Pathways of Spread of Anorectal Abscess

The anorectal abscess can spread through the following pathways:

A. ***Local or superficial spread:*** The infection starts in the anal glands or crypts in the submucosal space and is followed by formation of an abscess. Usually, the abscess bursts on its own. Sometimes, the abscess may extend into the intersphincteric space, perianal space or ischiorectal fossa due to ramifications of the anal glands (Fig. 6.2).

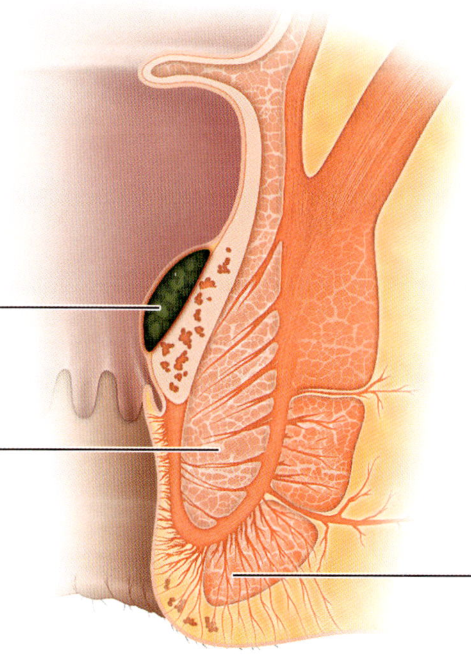

Fig. 6.2: Submucosal abscess

B. ***Intersphincteric spread:*** The infection can spread along the intersphincteric space. A downward extension from an intersphincteric abscess forms a perianal abscess, and an upward extension results in a supralevator abscess. A low or high intersphincteric fistula may follow (Fig. 6.3A and B).

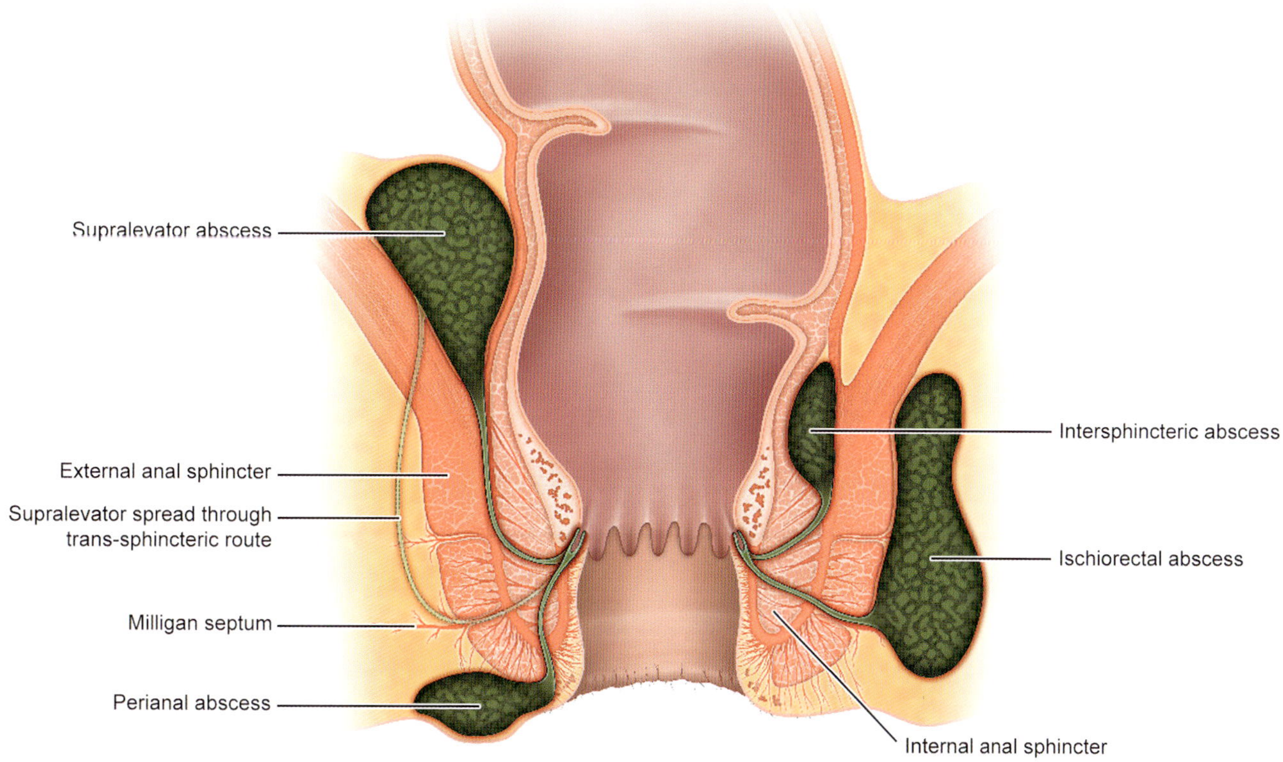

Fig. 6.3A: Pathways of the spread of abscesses

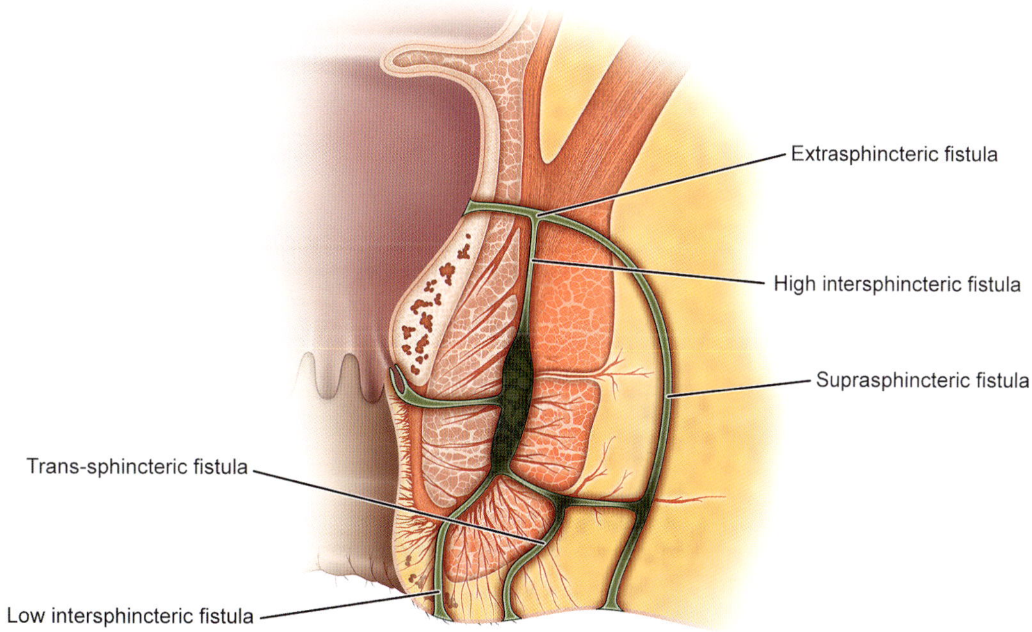

Fig. 6.3B: Correlation between fistulas and the abscesses

C. ***Trans-sphincteric spread*** occurs when the infection breaches the anal sphincter complex, extending the abscess through the sphincter muscles into the ischiorectal space. A trans-sphincteric fistula may follow, which may be low or high, depending on the extent of the external anal sphincter involved (Fig. 6.4A and B).

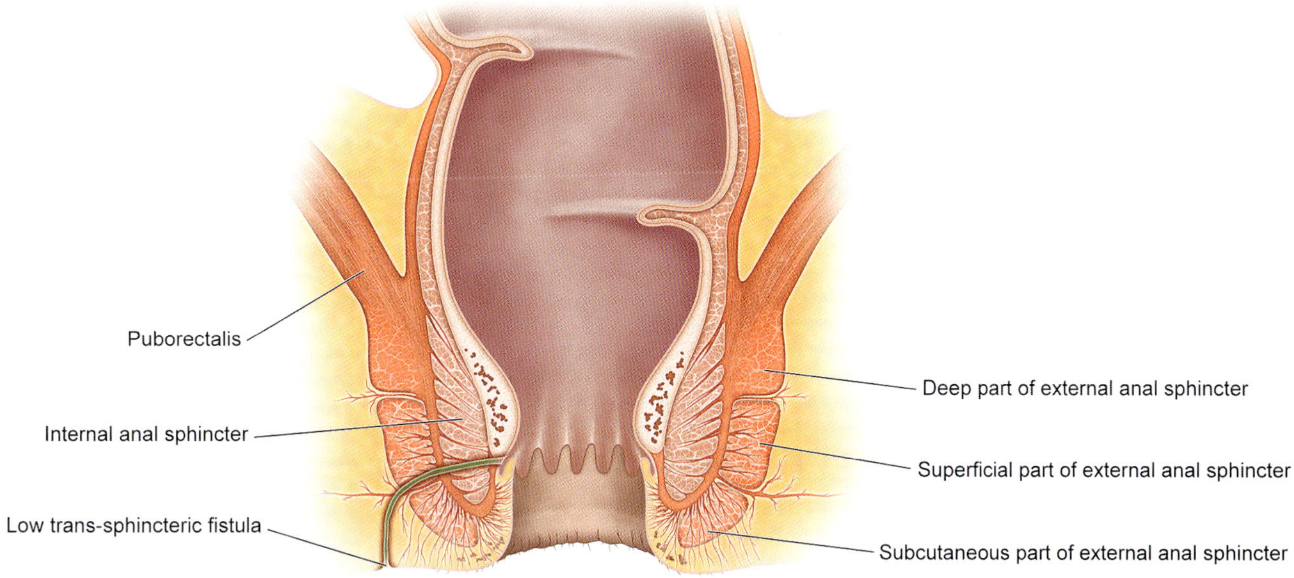

Fig. 6.4A: Low trans-sphincteric fistula

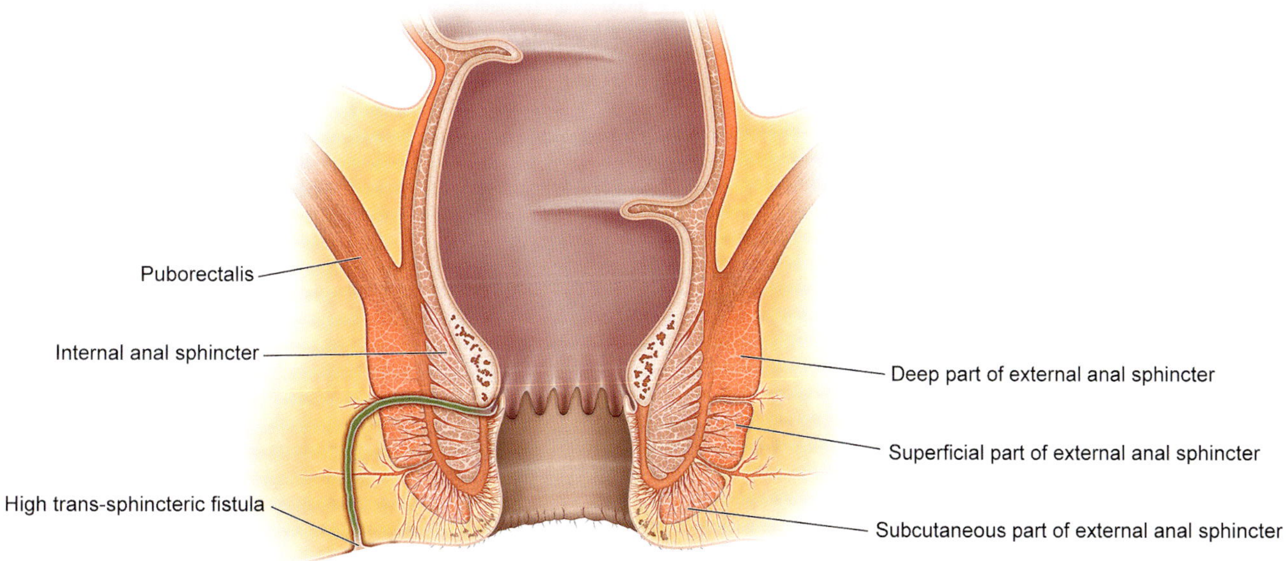

Fig. 6.4B: High trans-sphincteric fistula

D. ***Anterior spread:*** An abscess may extend through the urogenital triangle after piercing the superficial and deep transverse perineal muscles leading to the formation of an anterior abscess (Fig. 6.5).

E. ***Posterior spread:*** The abscess spreads to the posterior space towards the sacrotuberous ligament and gluteus maximus (Fig. 6.6). The resultant fistula opening may be in the gluteal region.

F. ***Horseshoe spread:*** The ischioanal fossae communicate through the deep postanal space. An abscess can spread through this space, forming a posterior horseshoe abscess (Fig. 6.6). An anterior spread may lead to an anterior horseshoe fistula.

G. ***Spread through perineal fascia:*** Fascial planes offer an anatomic pathway for the infection to the travel from the superficial to deep spaces. Rarely, the abscess and fistula may penetrate the fascia and present as an opening in the abdominal cavity or the medial aspect of the thigh (Fig. 6.5).

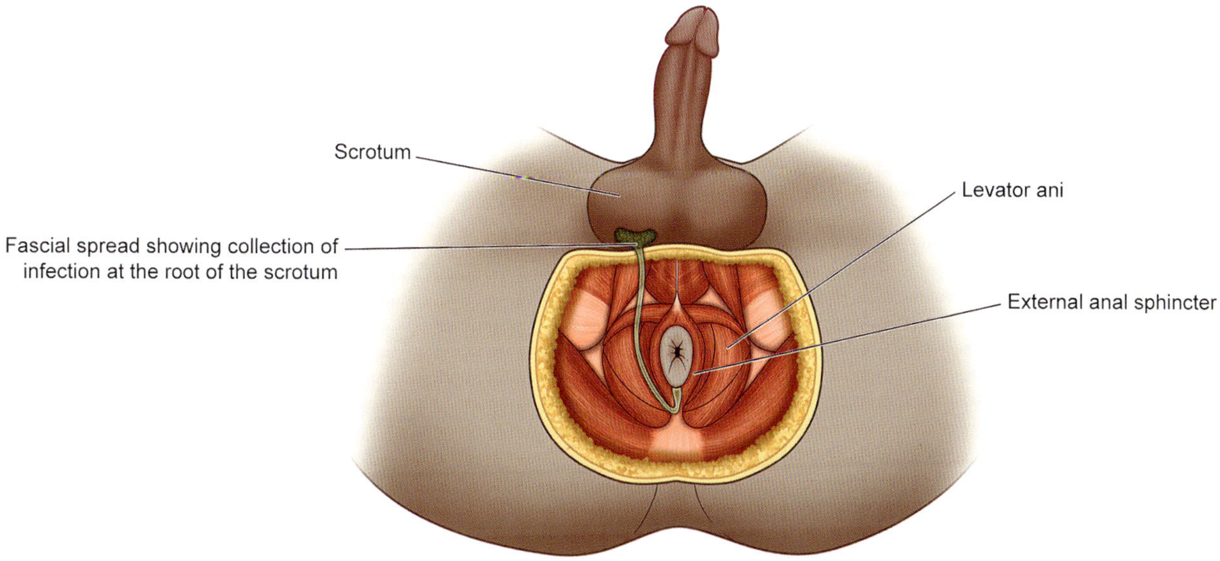

Fig. 6.5: Anterior and fascial spread of abscess

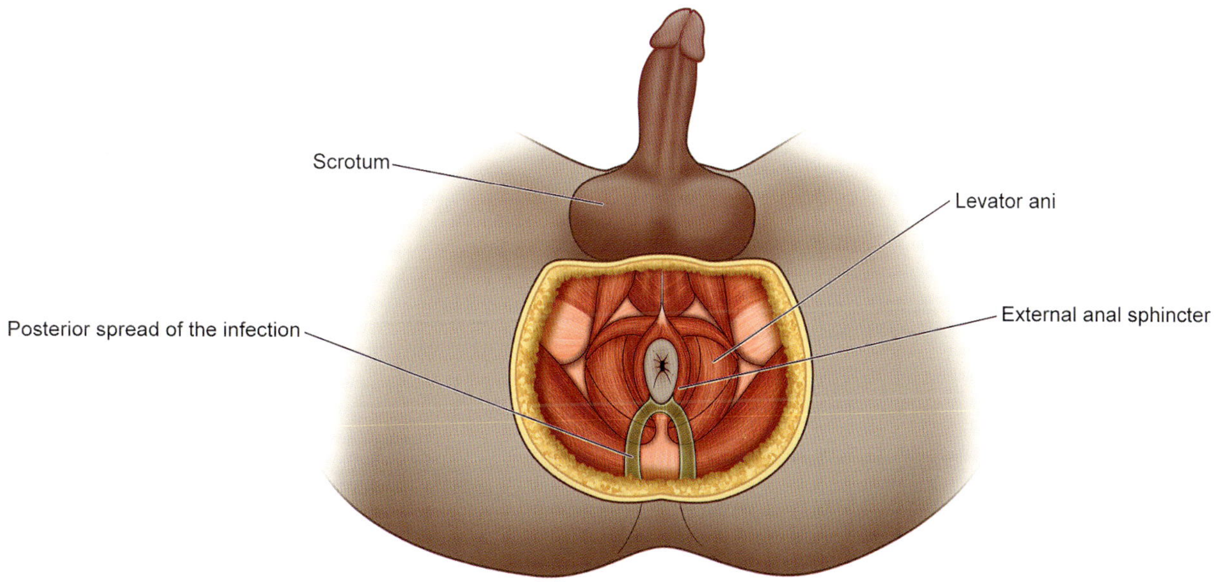

Fig. 6.6: Posterior and horseshoe spread

Spread through Anal Canal Musculature and Correlation between Abscesses and Fistulas

Intersphincteric Spread

- Intersphincteric space is the most potential space from where the infection can spread. The space is present between the internal and the external anal sphincter (Fig. 6.7A).
- Abscesses or fistulas can extend upward between the internal and the external sphincter muscles along the main longitudinal muscle bundle. This displaces the external sphincter muscles outward and allows the abscess or fistula to enter the anal canal through the internal sphincter along a longitudinal muscle bundle.
- The infection in this space can remain confined to form an intersphincteric abscess (Fig. 6.7B and C).

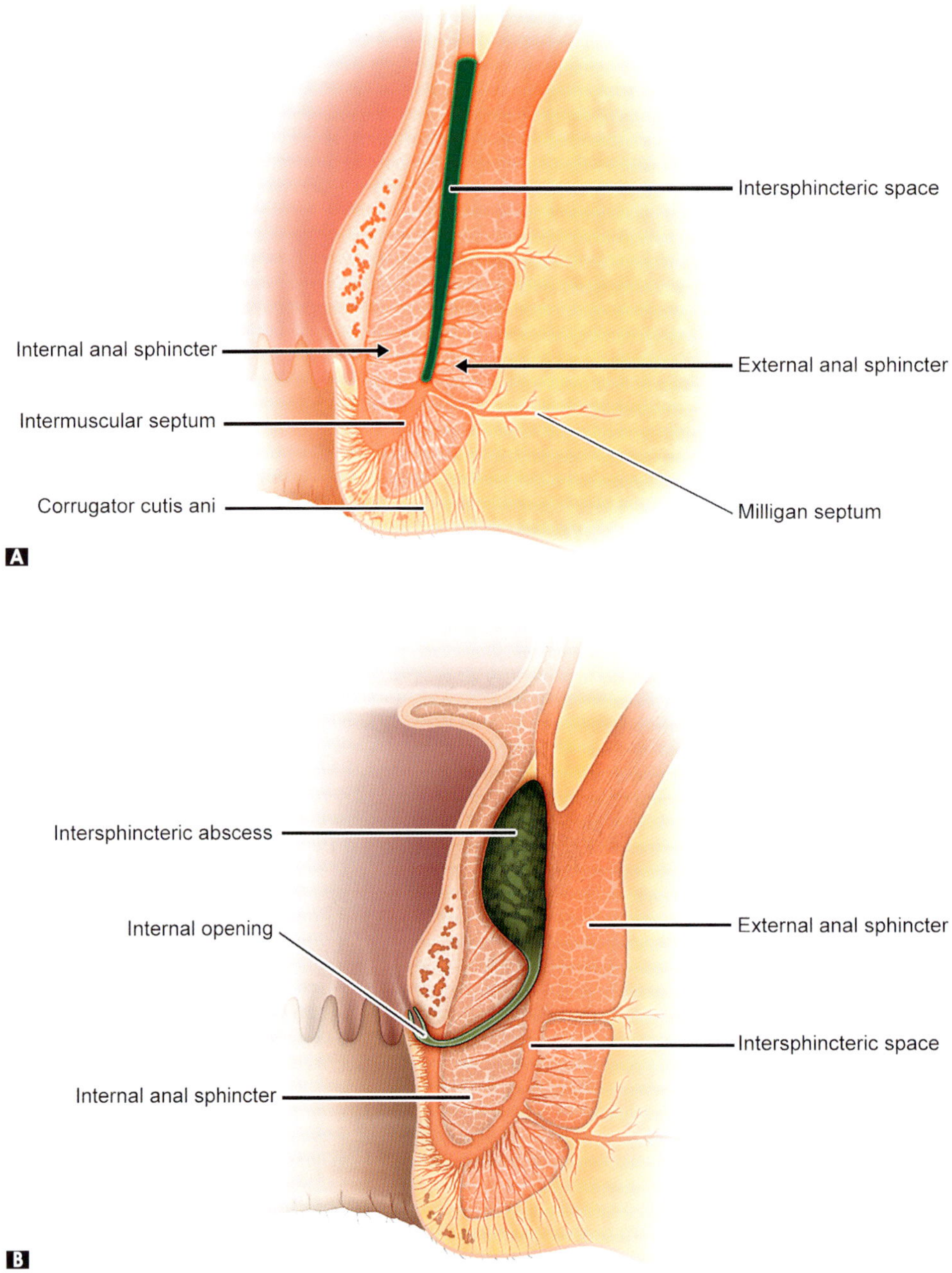

Fig. 6.7: (A) Intersphincteric space; (B) Intersphincteric abscess

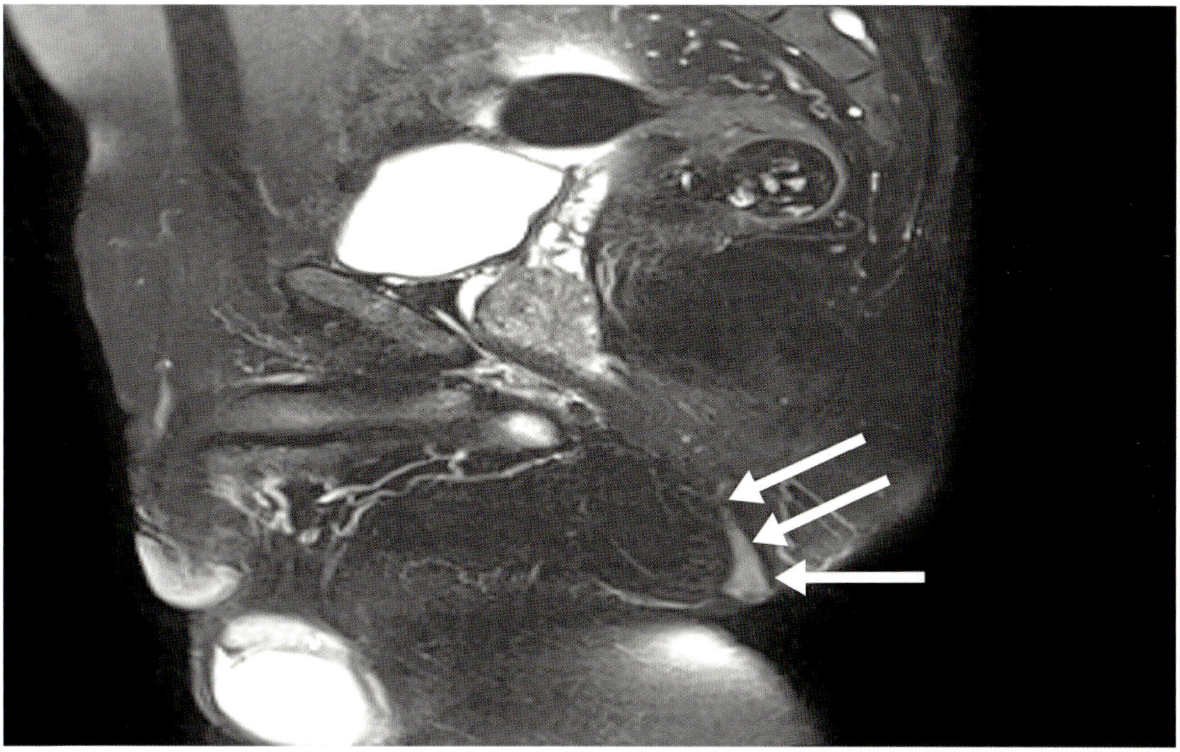

Fig. 6.7C: MRI images showing intersphincteric spread (*Courtesy:* Dr GS Bholla)

- Since most ramifications of the anal glands run caudally, a downward extension through the intersphincteric space leads to a perianal abscess (Fig. 6.7D and E).
- Because of the upward continuity of the intersphincteric space towards the levators, the infection can travel to the supralevator space to form a supralevator abscess (Fig. 6.7D).
- A posterior spread through the intersphincteric space can form an intersphincteric horseshoe abscess (refer to horseshoe abscesses Fig. 6.20A and B).

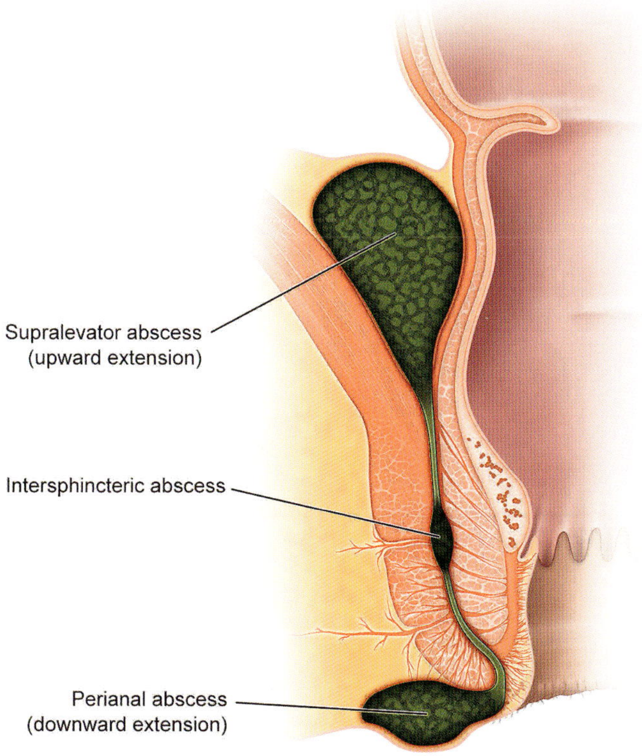

D

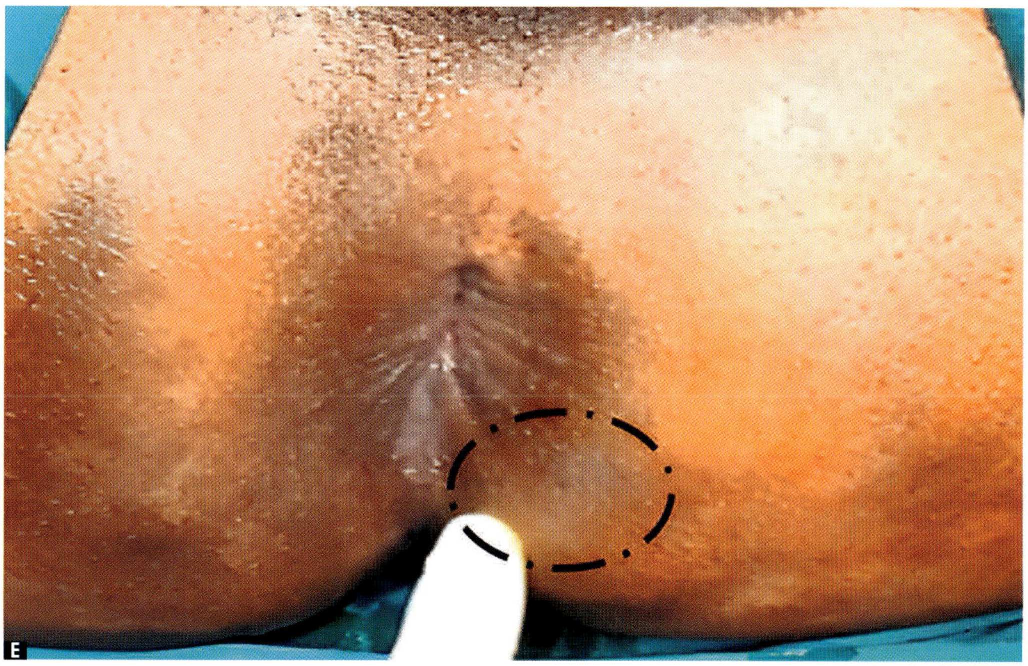

E

Fig. 6.7D and E: (D) Spread of infection from the intersphincteric space (downwards to form a perianal abscess and upwards towards levators to form a supralevator abscess); (E) Clinical presentation of perianal abscess

Correlation between intersphincteric abscess and intersphincteric fistulas

- The most common type of anorectal fistula is the intersphincteric, which originates in the intersphincteric space. It typically follows a straight course, extending from the anal canal to an external opening near the anus (Fig. 6.8A and B).

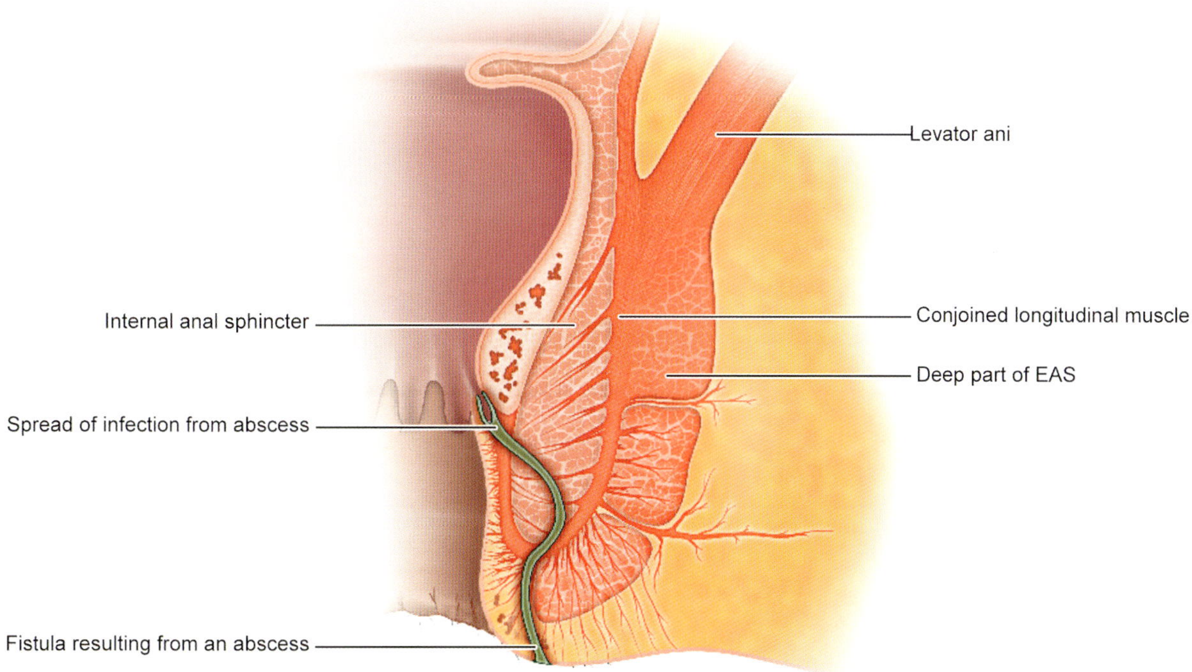

Fig. 6.8A: Formation of intersphincteric fistula (type A1)

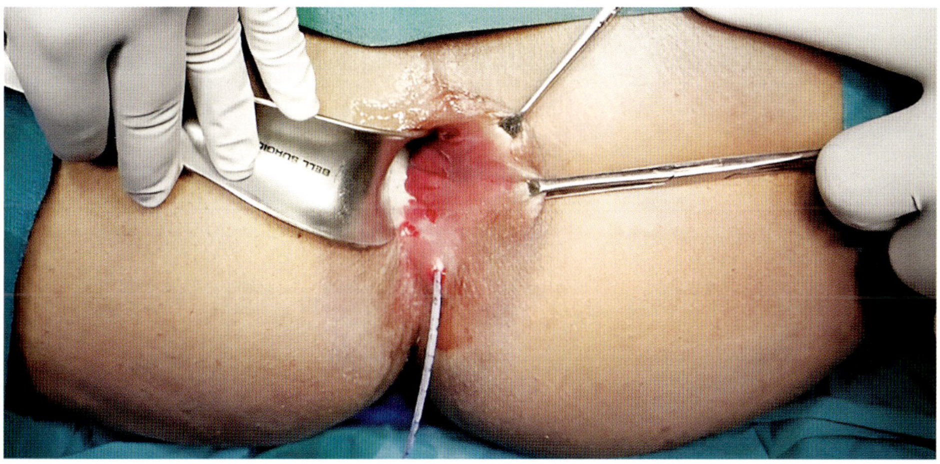

Fig. 6.8B: Clinical presentation of intersphincteric fistula

- A chronic intersphincteric infection may lead to type A2 or A3 fistulas (Fig. 6.9A and B). The type A3 fistula has two internal openings, one at the dentate line (origin of abscess) and the second above the dentate line, as shown in Fig. 6.9C. The second internal opening is as a result of intersphincteric extension, opening in the distal part of the rectum.

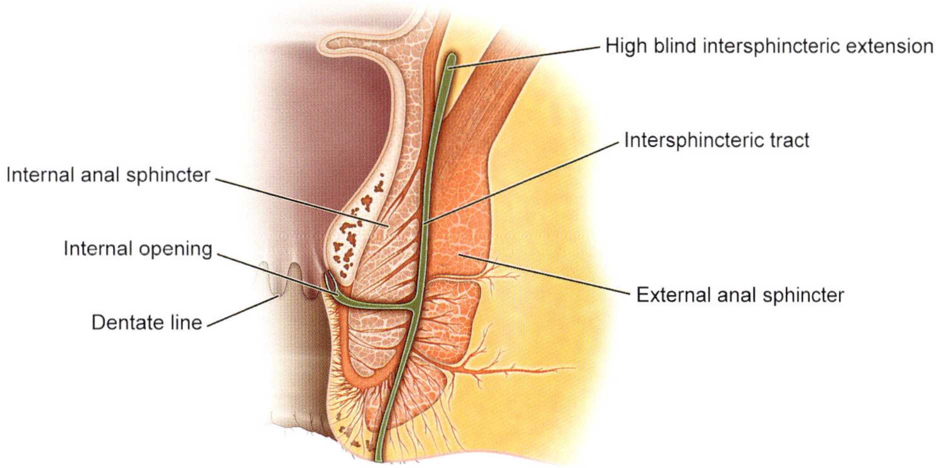

Fig. 6.9A: Intersphincteric fistula following intersphincteric abscess (type A2)

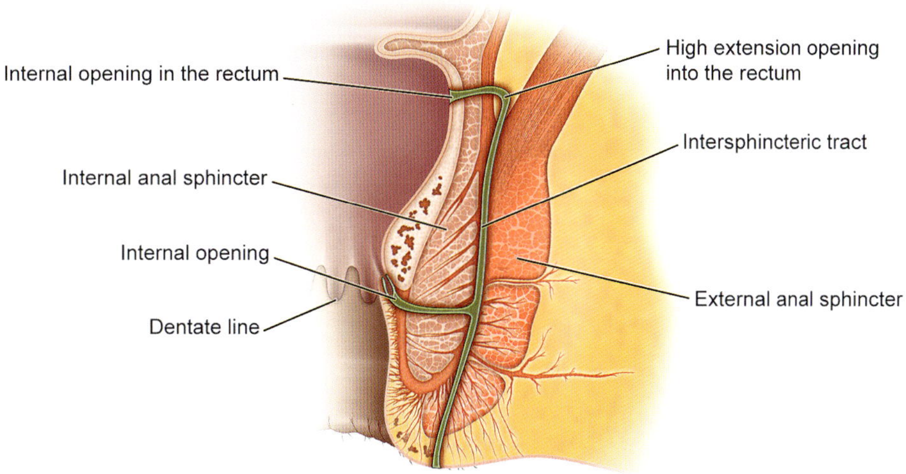

Fig. 6.9B: Intersphincteric fistula following intersphincteric abscess—type A3. The upward extension opens into the distal rectum

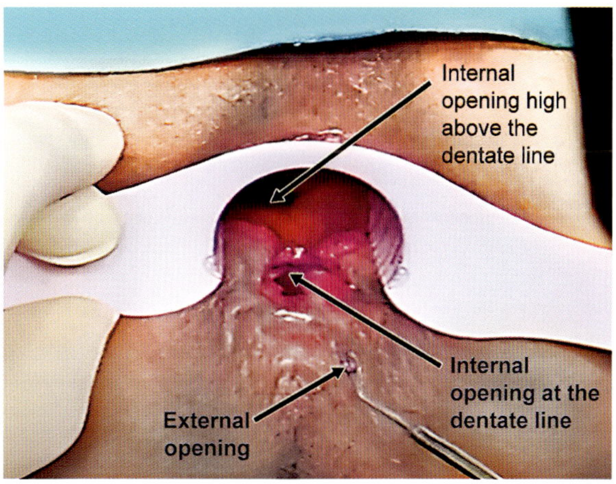

Fig. 6.9C: Internal openings at and above the dentate line

- The upward extension of an intersphincteric abscess may present as an intersphincteric fistula without an external opening, as shown in Fig. 6.10A and B (type A4 tract).

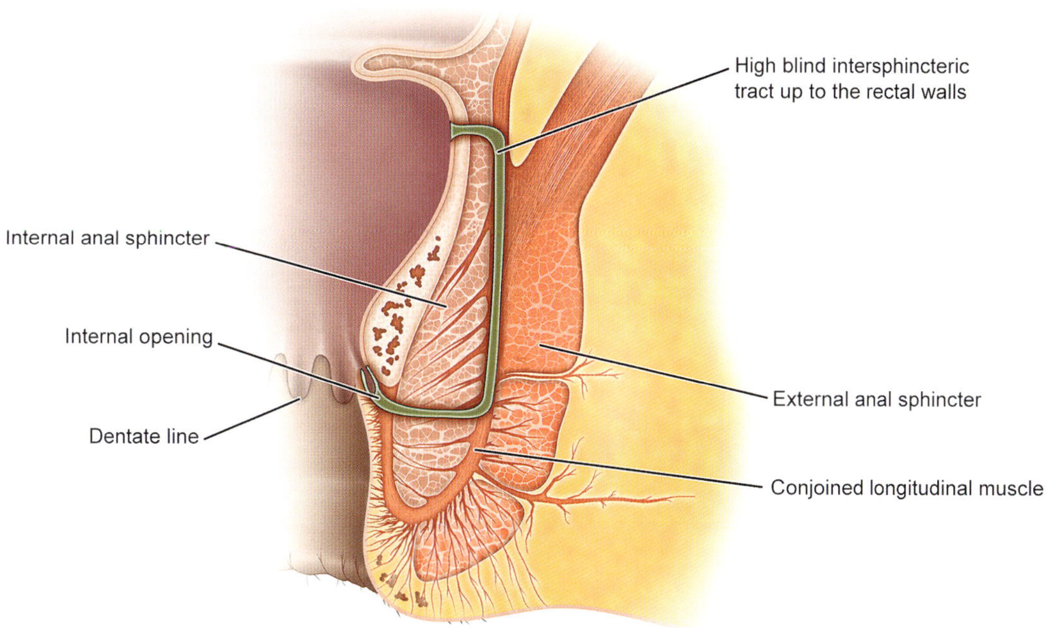

Fig. 6.10A: Intersphincteric fistula following intersphincteric abscess—type A4

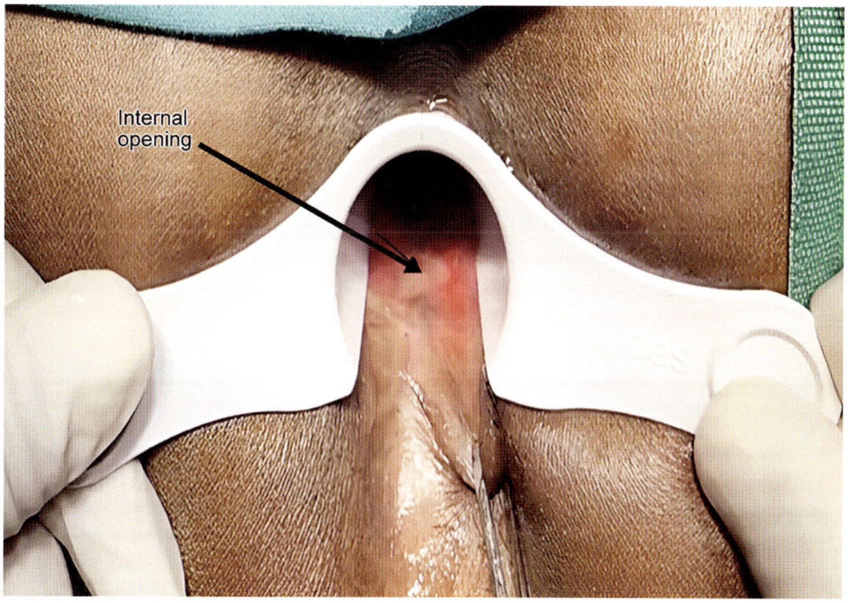

Fig. 6.10B: Clinical presentation of intersphincteric fistula type A4. The internal opening can be seen at 6 o'clock at the dentate line. There is no external opening

- A supralevator extension forms type A5 of the fistula, as shown in Fig. 6.10C. Since there is no downwards extension towards the anal verge, there are no clinical signs of fistula.
- An extension of a pelvic infection extends downwards to reach the intersphincteric plane and form type A6 intersphincteric fistula as shown in Fig. 6.10D.

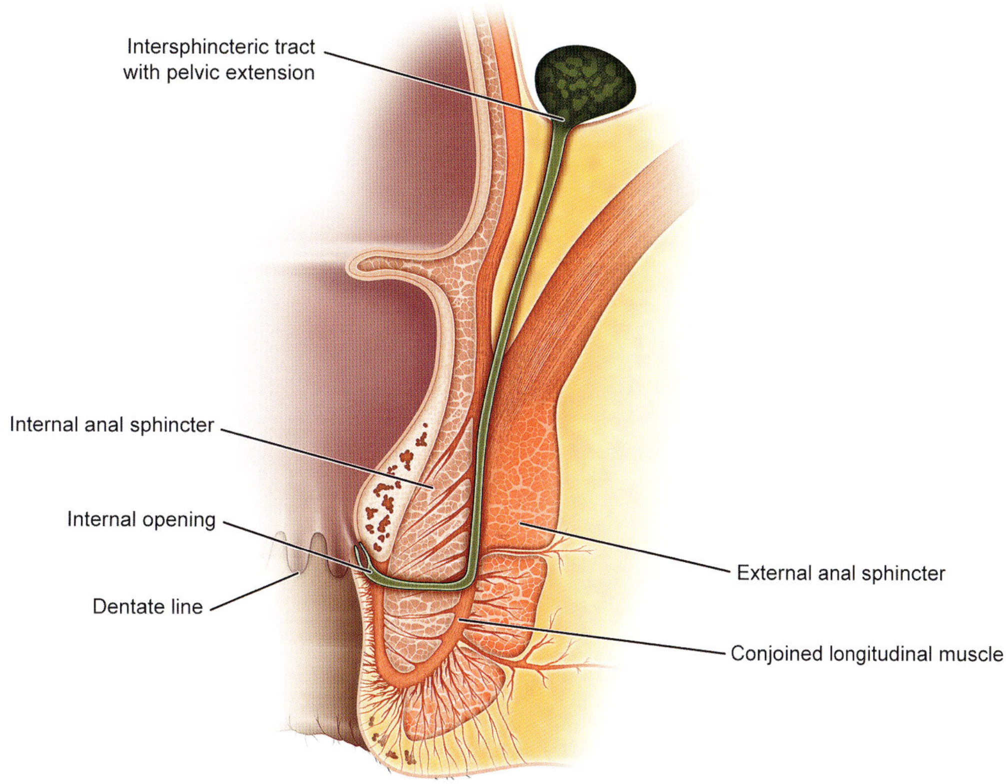

Fig. 6.10C: Intersphincteric fistula formed after supralevator extension—type A5

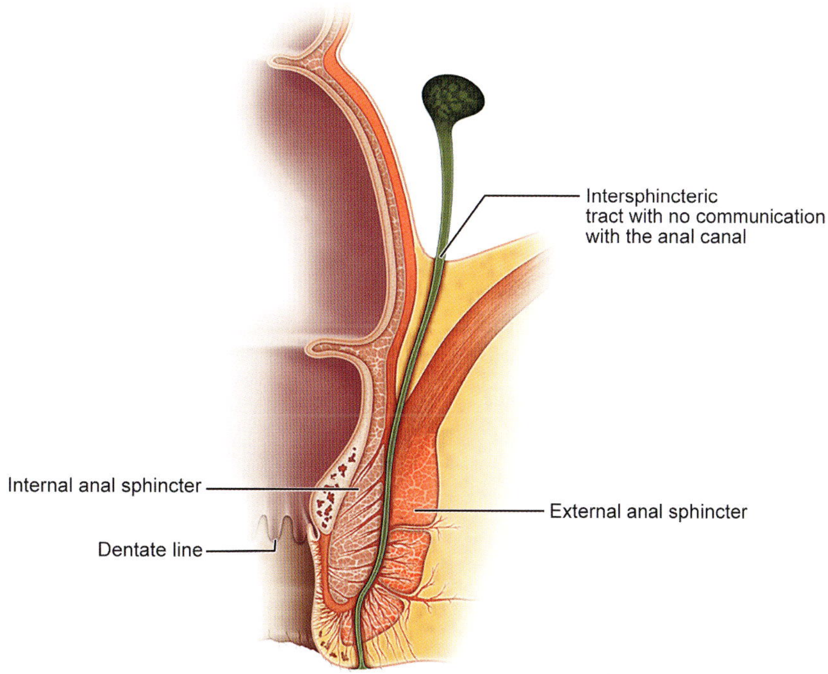

Fig. 6.10D: Intersphincteric fistula—type A6

Trans-sphincteric Spread

- The spread occurs when the infection crosses the internal and external anal sphincters and reaches the ischiorectal space (Fig. 6.11A and B).

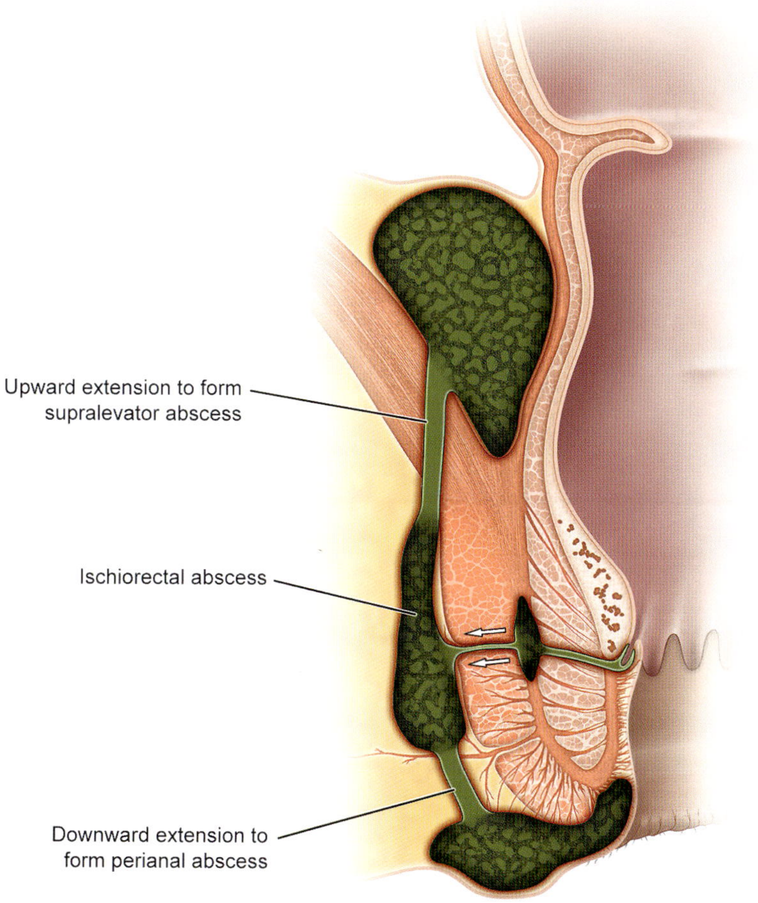

Fig. 6.11A: Diagrammatic representation of the infection crossing the internal and external anal sphincters and reaching the ischiorectal space to form an ischiorectal abscess

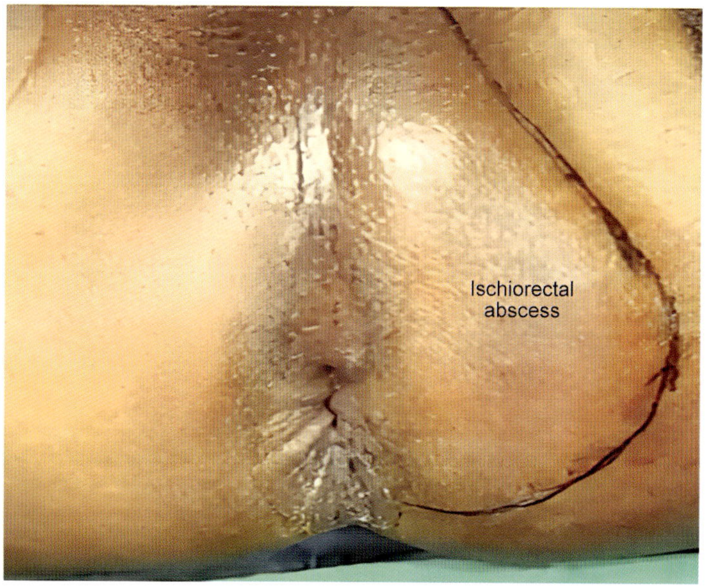

Fig. 6.11B: Clinical presentation of an ischiorectal abscess. The outer extent of the abscess has been demarcated with a marker

Correlation between Trans-sphincteric Abscess and Fistula

- Once a trans-sphincteric abscess (ischiorectal abscess) is formed, it may result in the formation of a trans-sphincteric fistula. This type of fistula crosses the external and internal anal sphincters and is referred to as type B1 (Fig. 6.12A and B).

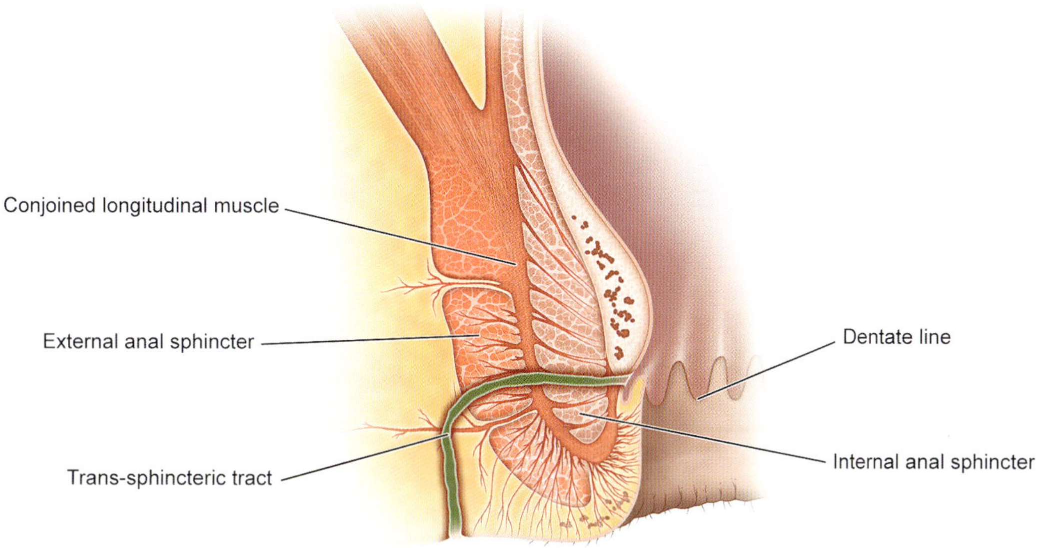

Fig. 6.12A: Diagrammatic representation of the formation of trans-sphincteric fistula

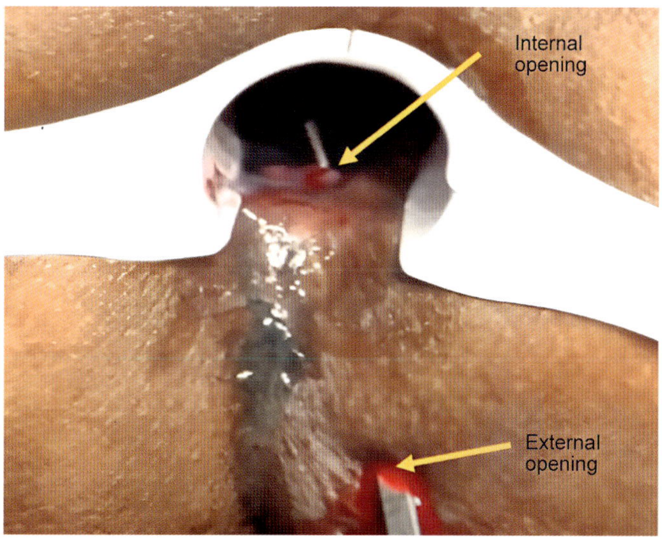

Fig. 6.12B: Clinical presentation of trans-sphincteric fistula. The probe can be seen coming out of the internal opening at 6 o'clock at the dentate line

- An extension can arise from the trans-sphincteric tract and progress upwards, giving rise to type B2 tract, as shown in Fig. 6.12C.

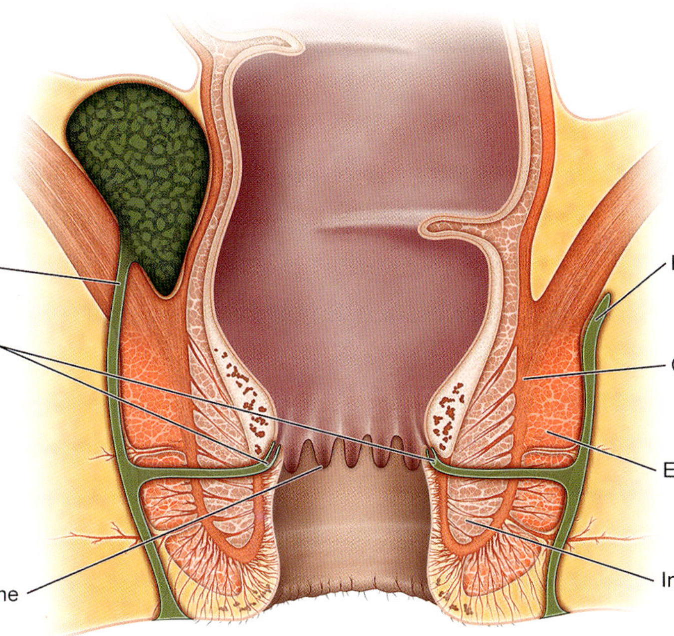

Fig. 6.12C: Trans-sphincteric fistula with extension type B2

- Another variation of the trans-sphincteric fistula may be present as an intersphincteric extension (Fig. 6.12D).
- Sometimes in a trans-sphincteric fistula, multiple external openings may be present with a single internal opening (Fig. 6.12E).

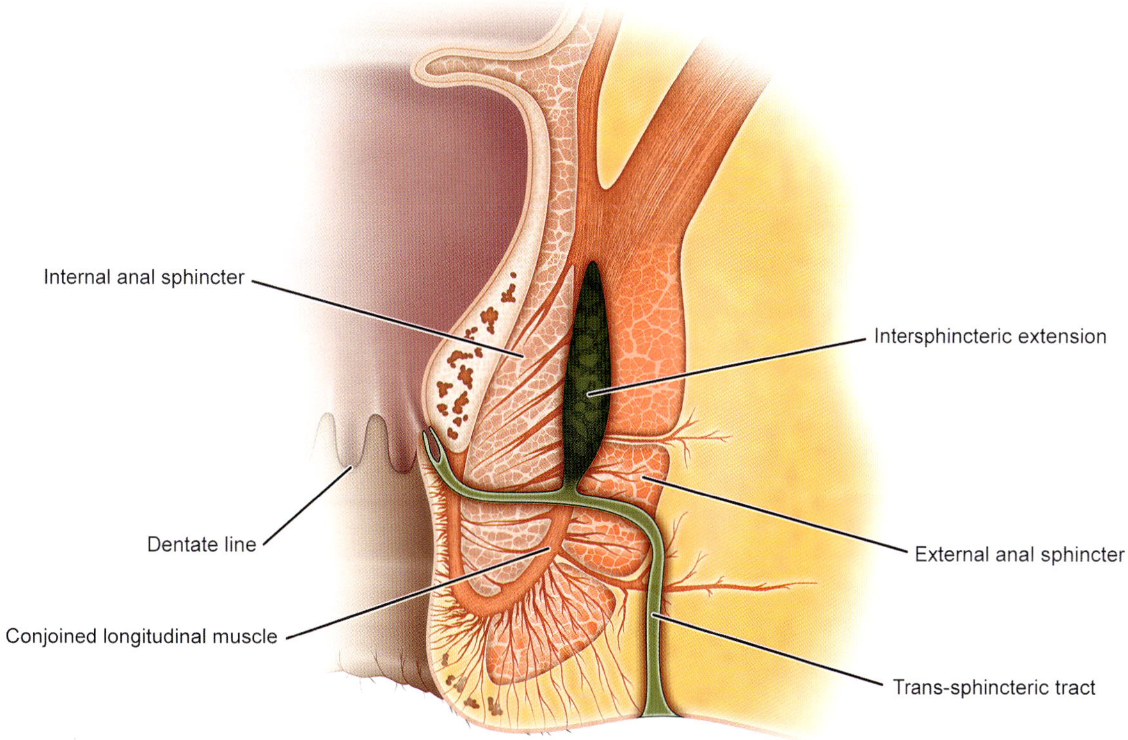

Fig. 6.12D: Trans-sphincteric fistula with intersphincteric extension

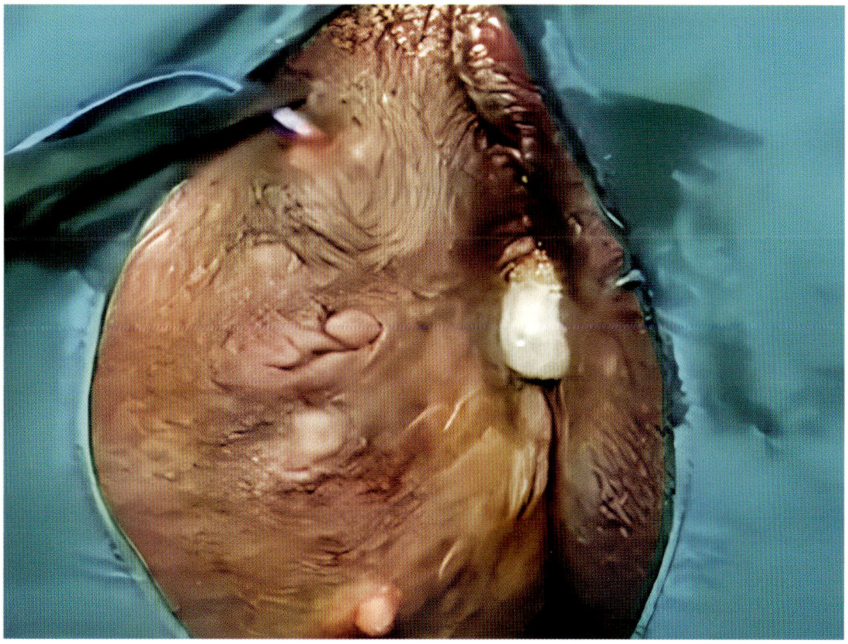

Fig. 6.12E: Clinical presentation of trans-sphincteric fistula with multiple external openings and a single internal opening

Spread to Infralevator Space

- The infection may spread through the deep part of the external anal sphincter and levator ani into the infralevator space. The abscess formed is an infralevator abscess (Fig. 6.13).

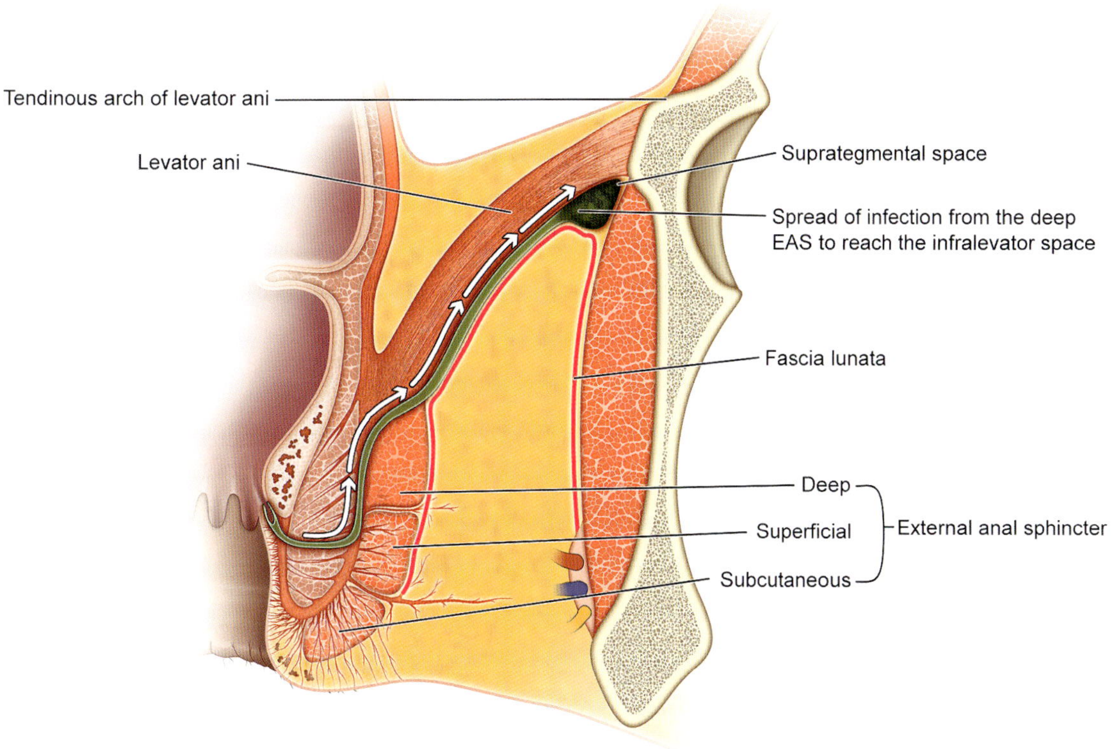

Fig. 6.13: Diagrammatic representation of the infection spreading through the deep part of the external anal sphincter and levator ani to the infralevator space to form an infralevator abscess. The arrows show the pathway of the spread of the abscess

Spread to the Supralevator Space

- The supralevator space is located above the levator ani (puborectalis) and is in close proximity to the pelvic cavity.
- An intersphincteric abscess can extend upwards, resulting in a supralevator abscess, as shown in Fig. 6.7D.
- An abscess from the ischiorectal and the infralevator space may pierce fascia lunata and infralevator fascia to form a supralevator abscess. The subsequent fistula formed is suprasphincteric. The suprasphincteric fistulas originate in the anal canal and extend upwards, passing above the sphincter complex (internal anal sphincter, external anal sphincter and puborectalis) before reaching the perianal region to form an external opening (Fig. 6.14A and B).

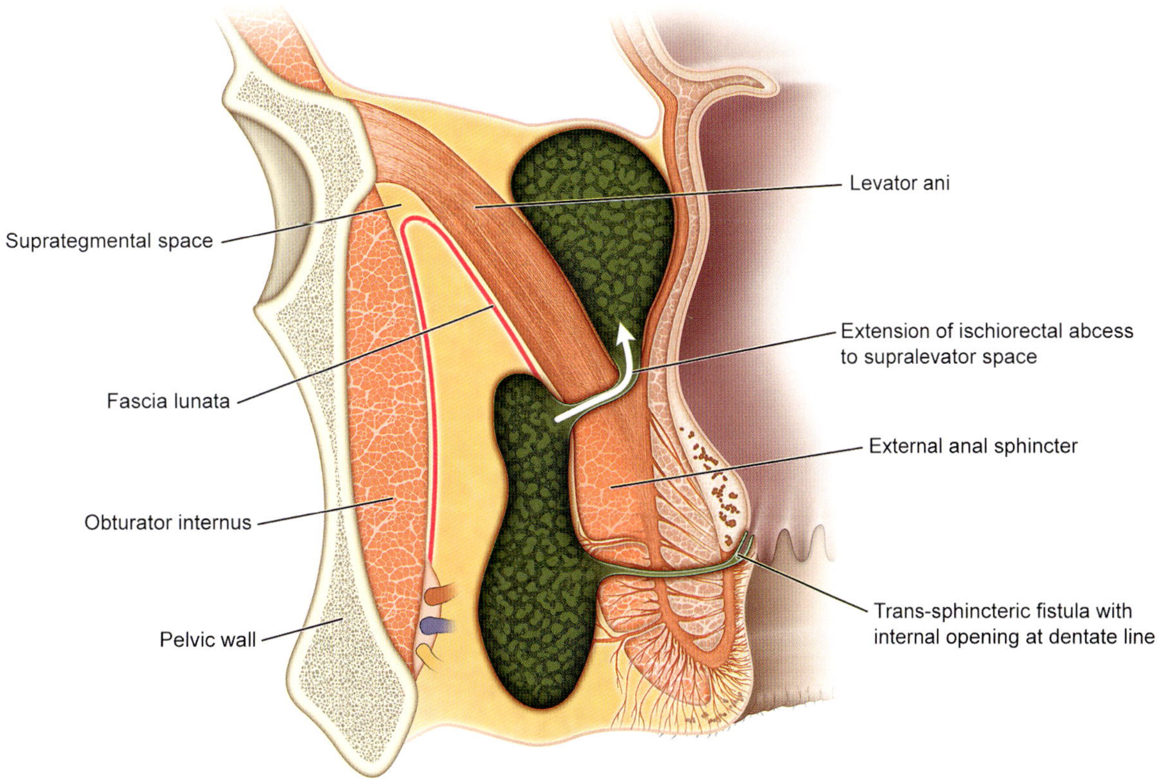

Fig. 6.14A: Diagrammatic representation of spread of an abscess piercing fascia lunata and infralevator fascia to form a supralevator abscess

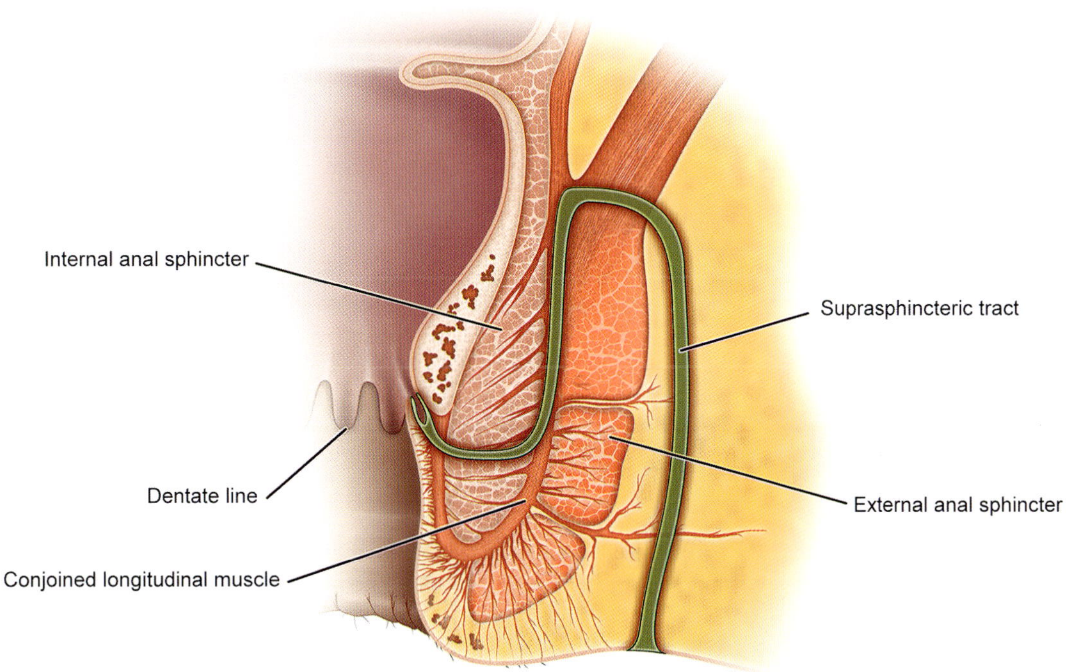

Fig. 6.14B: Suprasphincteric fistula tract

- A downward extension from the pelvis can also lead to a supralevator abscess. The spread occurs through the pelvic fascia (Fig. 6.14C).

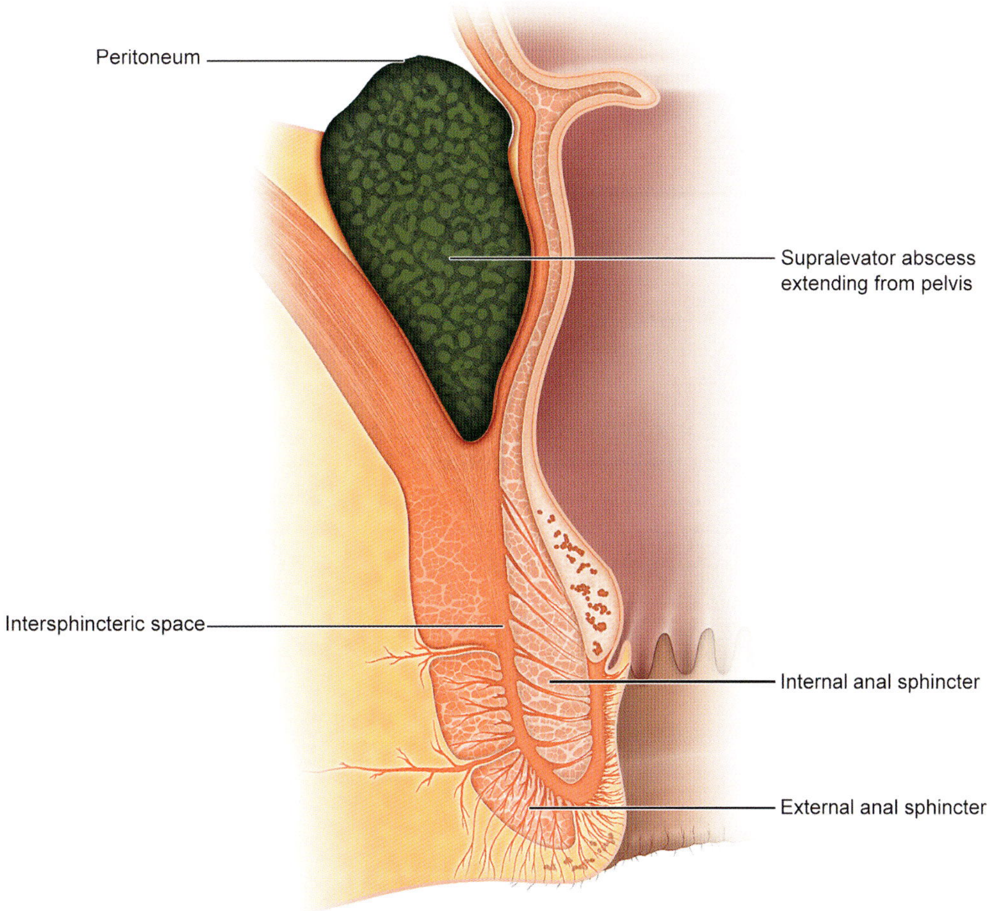

Fig. 6.14C: Spread from pelvic infection

Extrasphincteric Spread

- The extrasphincteric spread does not involve the anal gland and is mainly of non-cryptoglandular origin. The extrasphincteric fistulas bypass the anal canal entirely. They connect the proximal rectum directly to the perianal region. This type of fistula is usually associated with Crohn's disease (Fig. 6.15A and B). Any trauma to the rectum can also lead to an extrasphincteric fistula. The exception is the tracts associated with an iatrogenic injury during probing or a surgical procedure (Fig. 6.15C).

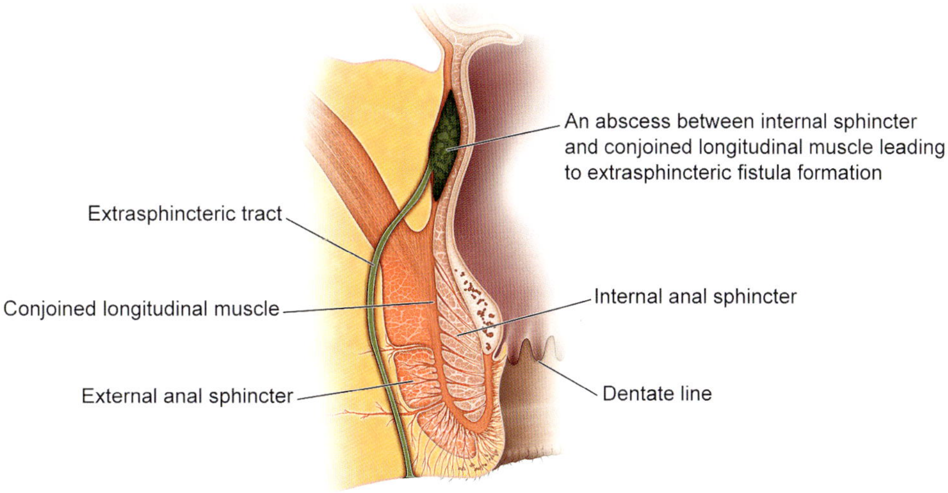

Fig. 6.15A: Crohn's abscess

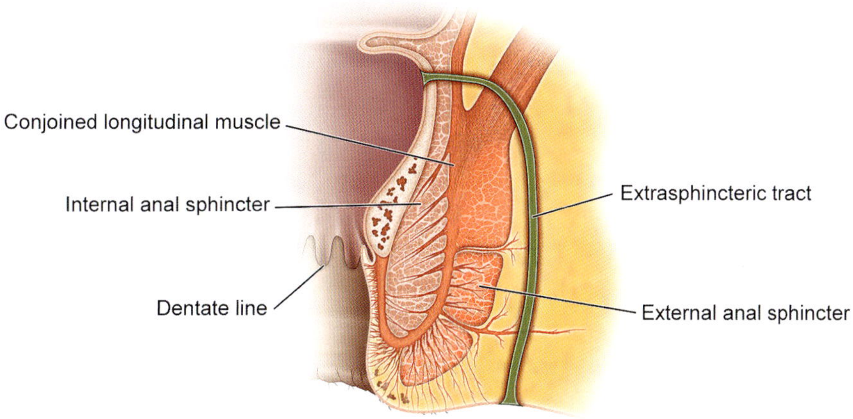

Fig. 6.15B: Extrasphincteric fistula bypassing the entire sphincter complex

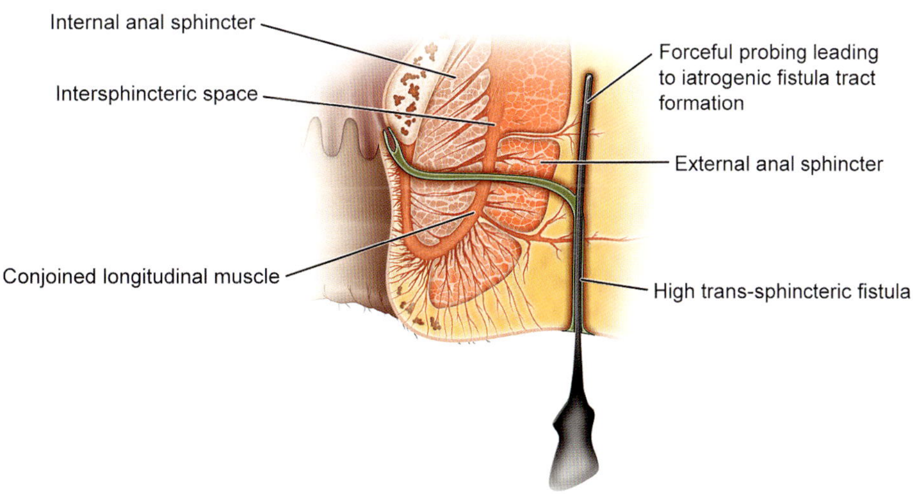

Fig. 6.15C: Forceful probing causing injury and forming an iatrogenic extrasphincteric fistula tract

Anterior Spread (Spread through perineal fascias)

The anterior spread occurs through the perineal fascias. The abscess may extend anteriorly to involve the medial aspect of the thigh, the labia in females, and the scrotum in males (Fig. 6.16A and B). Once the abscess bursts, a fistula may form.

- The fascias of the perineum encircle the anal canal. These layers include the superficial perineal fascia (Colles' fascia), the inferior layer of the urogenital diaphragm (perineal membrane), and the deep perineal fascia (superior layer of the urogenital diaphragm). Below the deep perineal fascia lies the pelvic diaphragm (levator ani muscles).

  As the anorectal abscess spreads, it might dissect through these planes and spread to other regions.

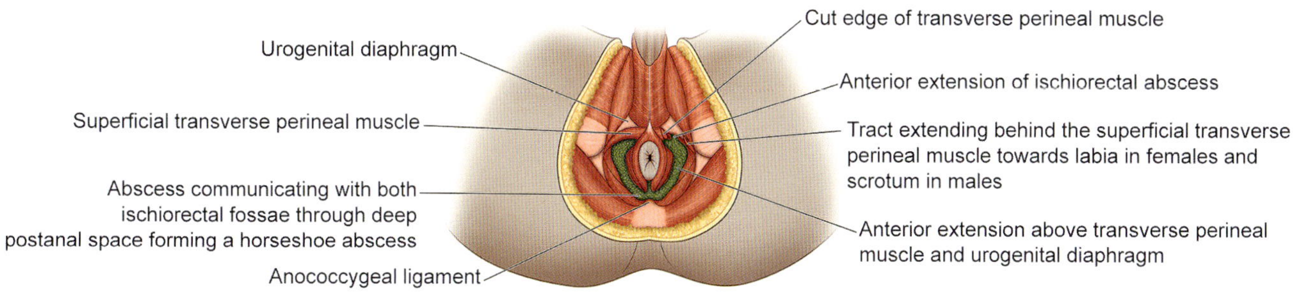

Fig. 6.16A: Anterior spread of the abscess

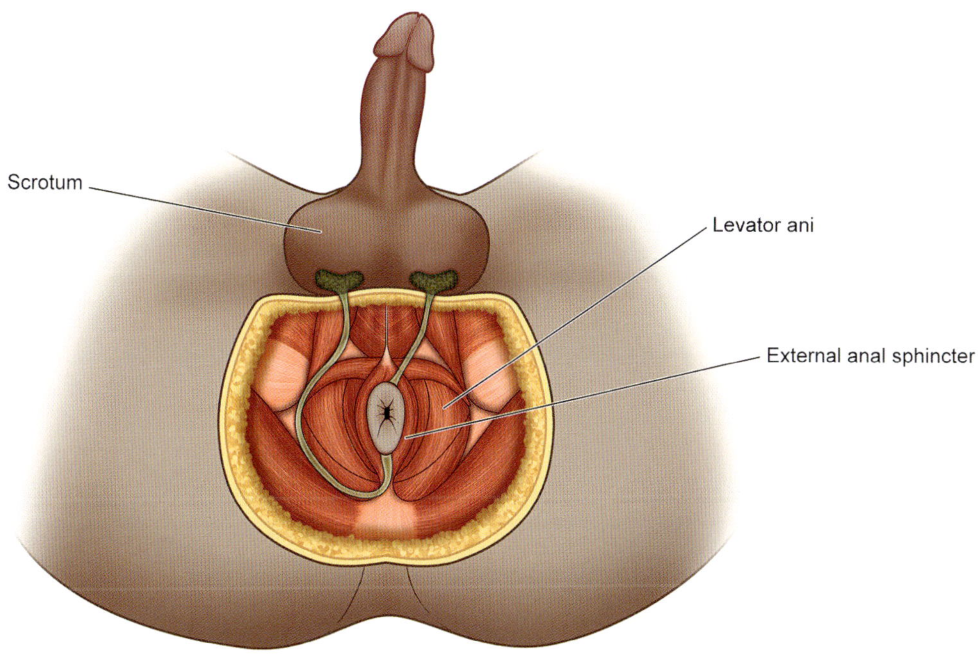

Fig. 6.16B: Diagrammatic representation of fistula formation after the anterior spread of infection. The infection can start at 6 or 12 o'clock and extend anteriorly

- As discussed in the anatomy of the perineum, the fascias play an essential role in forming two crucial spaces, the superficial and the deep perineal space. Since the Colles' fascia of the superficial space lacks the anterior boundary, it becomes a potent pathway of anterior spread (Fig. 6.17).

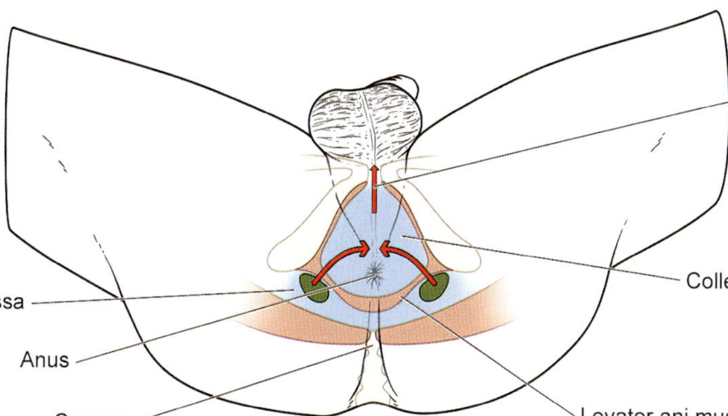

Fig. 6.17: Spread of the abscess through fascias. The arrows show the pathway of the spread of the abscess anteriorly through Colles' fascia

- When the infection spreads anteriorly, it can reach the superficial perineal space and pass through the superficial and deep transverse perineal muscle. In males, an anterior abscess may form at the root of the scrotum, penoscrotal junction or inguinal region (Fig. 6.18A and B). In females, the anterior extension is towards the labia majora.

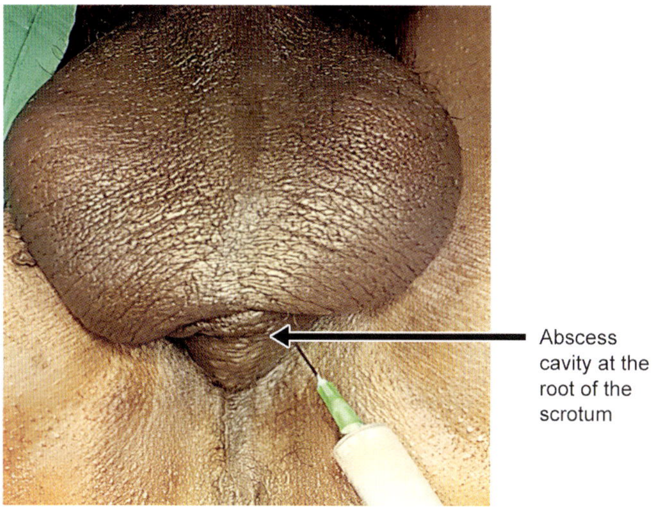

Fig. 6.18A: Abscess cavity at the root of the scrotum (anterior spread in males)

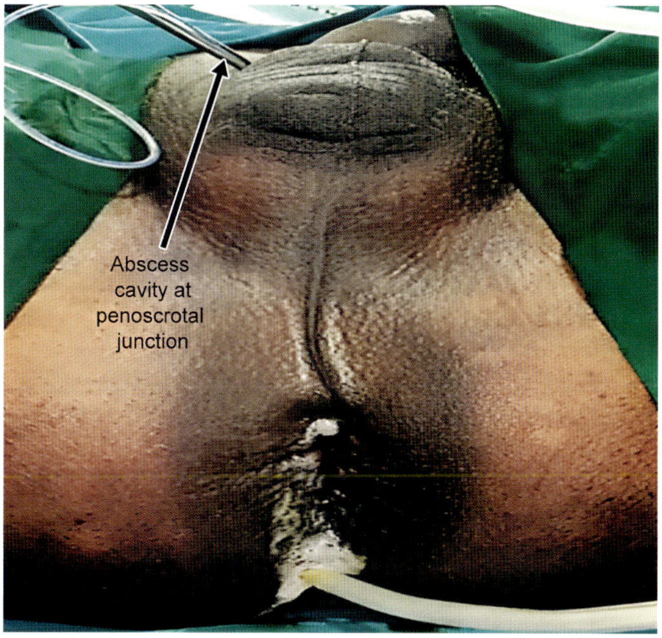

Fig. 6.18B: Abscess cavity at the penoscrotal junction (anterior spread in males)

- As the superficial perineal space is devoid of an anterior boundary, the pus can cross Colles' fascia and Scarpa's fascia to form an opening in the anterior abdominal wall (Fig. 6.19A and B).
- The superficial fascia of the anterior abdominal wall (Scarpa's fascia) is continuous with the deep fascia of the thigh (fascia lata). The pus can dissect through this plane and spread to the medial aspect of the thigh (Fig. 6.19A and B).

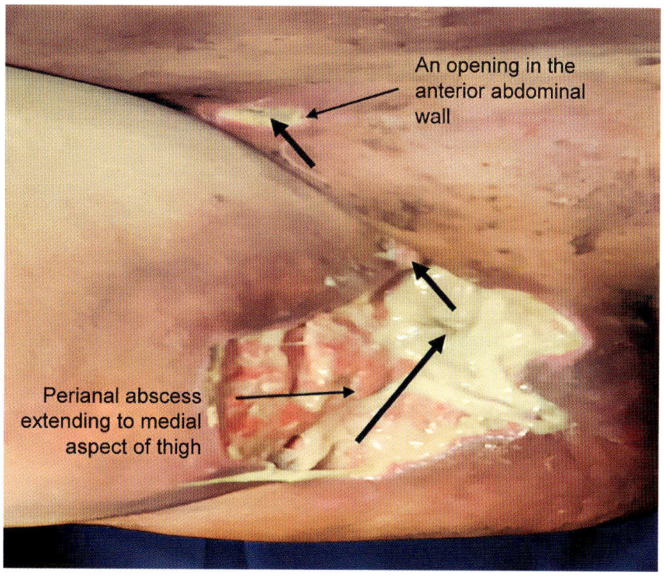

Fig. 6.19A: Perianal abscess spreading towards the medial aspect of the thigh and anterior abdominal wall

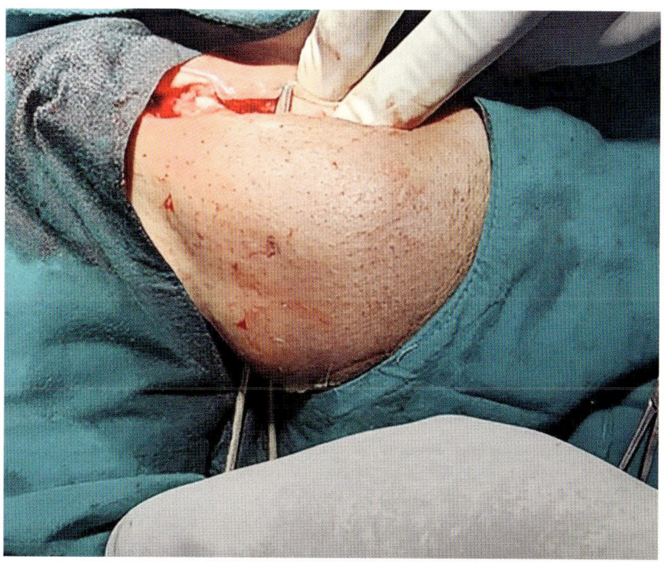

Fig. 6.19B: Blunt artery inserted from the perineum to show communication with the anterior abdominal wall

Posterior Spread

- The posterior spread occurs towards the sacrotuberous ligament and the gluteus maximus (Fig. 6.20).
- The resultant abscess formed is in the gluteal region.

Spread to Deep Postanal Space

- Most anal glands are present posteriorly. Once the glands get infected, the infection can spread posteriorly into the deep postanal space below the anococcygeal ligament (Fig. 6.21).
- The spread through the deep postanal space is the most common cause of a posterior horseshoe abscess and fistula formation.

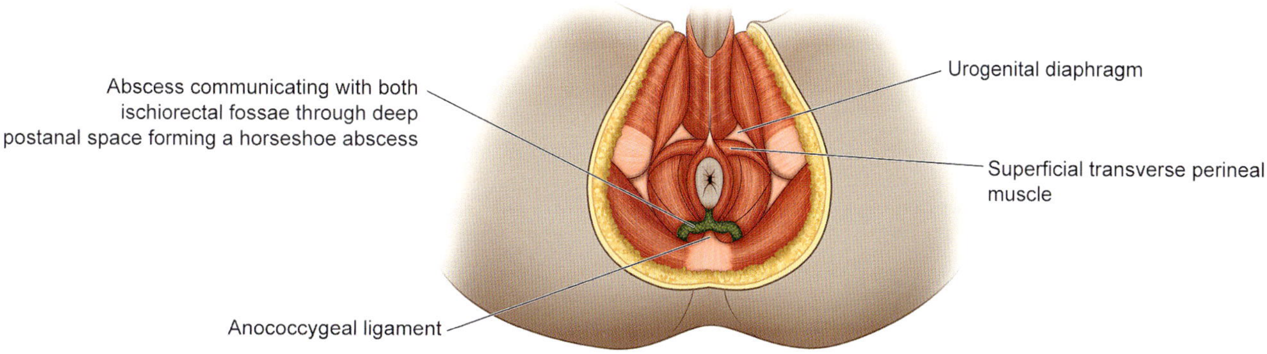

Fig. 6.20: Posterior spread of abscess

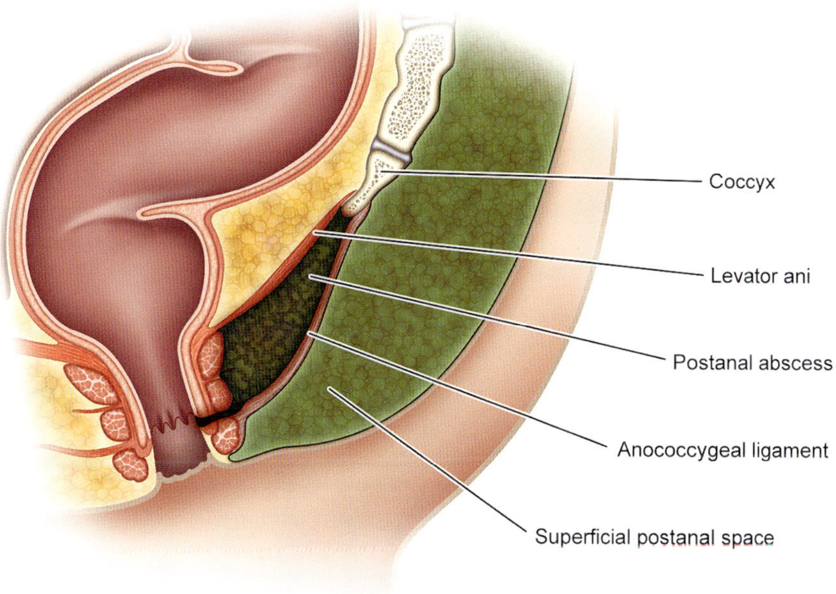

Fig. 6.21: The deep postanal space abscess

Horseshoe Abscess and Fistula

The horseshoe abscesses usually spread posteriorly and circumferentially (Fig. 6.22).

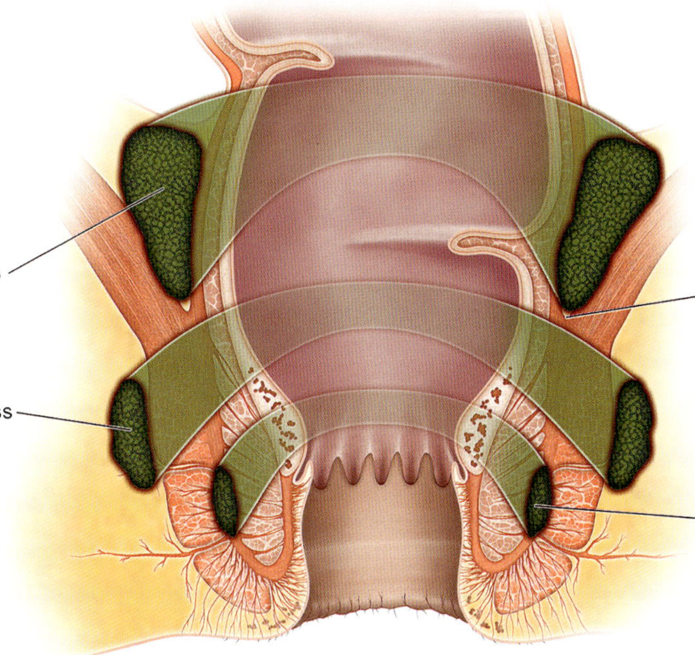

Fig. 6.22: Pathways of horseshoe abscesses

- The circumferential spread into the intersphincteric space may lead to a horseshoe intersphincteric abscess. The subsequent fistula formed may be of A4 type (Fig. 6.23A and B).

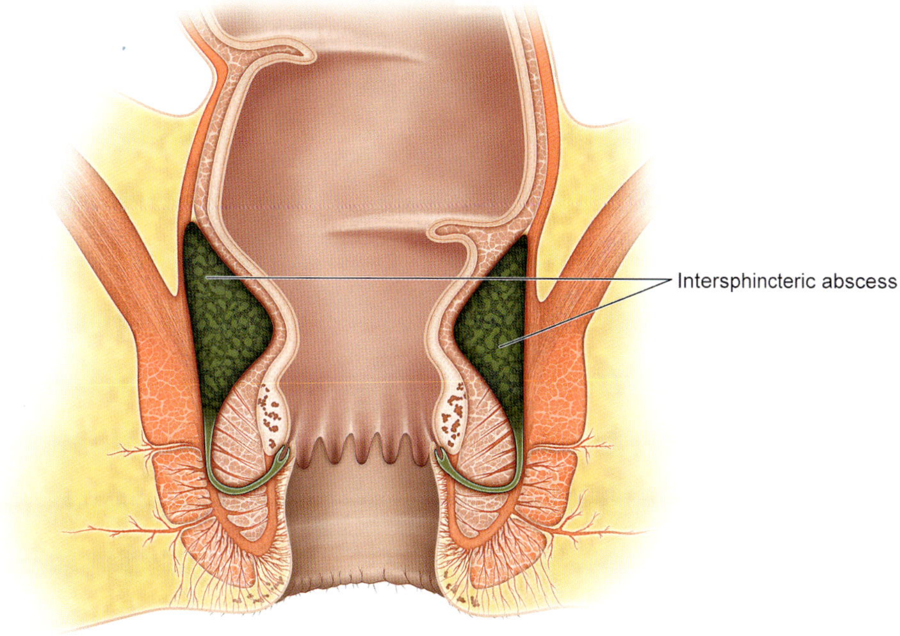

Fig. 6.23A: Diagrammatic representation of a horseshoe intersphincteric abscess

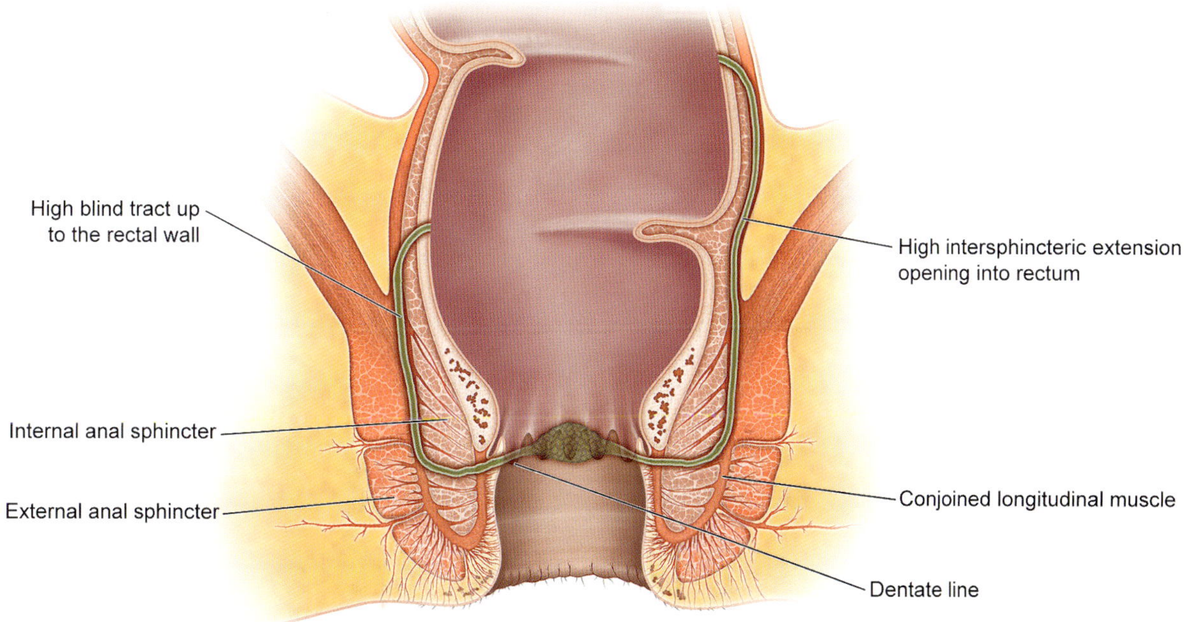

Fig. 6.23B: A4 type of fistula formation

- As the deep postanal space communicates with the ischiorectal fossae on either side, an abscess may spread posteriorly and circumferentially, forming an ischiorectal horseshoe abscess (Fig. 6.24).
- Similarly, a posterior spread may lead to the formation of a horseshoe suprasphincteric abscess (Fig. 6.22).

Retrorectal Spread

An untreated anorectal abscess between the internal anal sphincter and the conjoined longitudinal muscle may rupture the longitudinal muscle above the level of puborectalis and form a retrorectal abscess. (Fig. 6.25). The abscess may spread through the pelvic fascia, which is continuous with the retrorectal fascia.

Conclusion

Early recognition and surgical intervention are crucial to prevent the spread of an abscess. A surgeon must be aware of the anal canal musculature and the fascias, which form potential pathways for the spread of the disease. Inappropriate management can lead to recurrence.

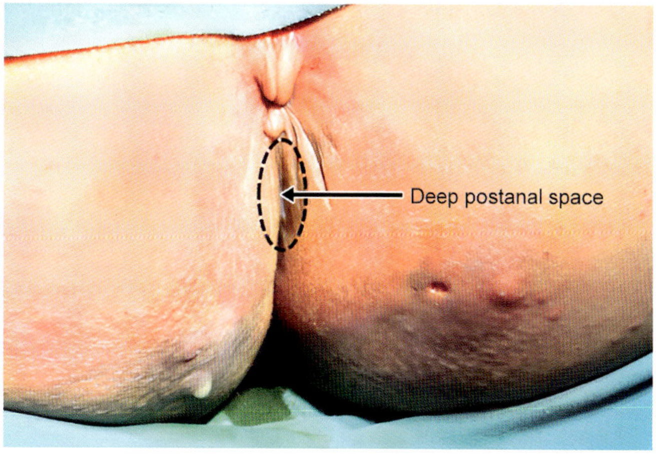

Fig. 6.24: Clinical presentation of horseshoe spread through deep postanal space

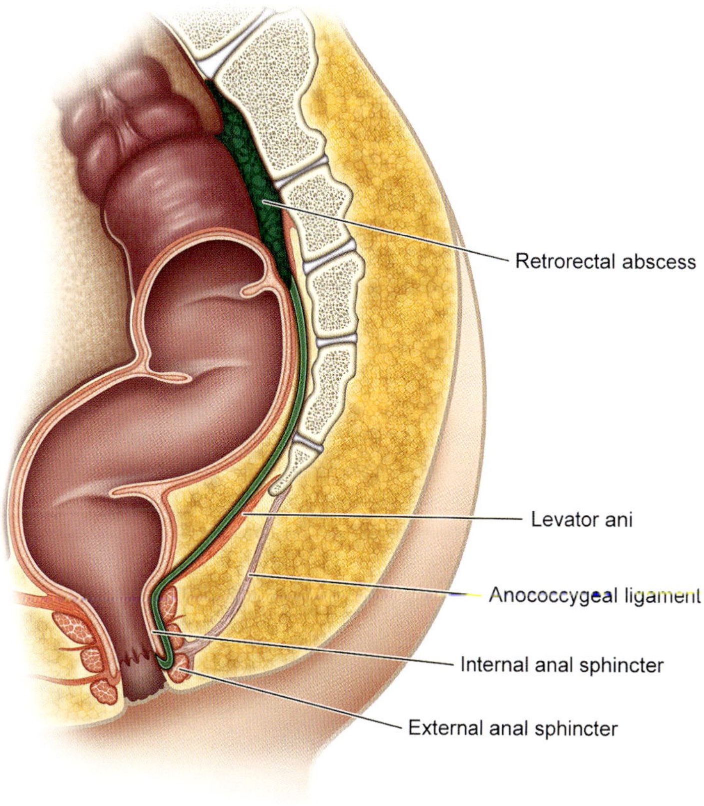

Fig. 6.25: Retrorectal spread of abscess

Further Reading

- Author: Andre Hebra, MD; Chief Editor: John Geibel, MD, MSc, DSc, AGAF. What is the Goodsall rule for the management of fistulas in the treatment of anorectal abscesses? July 24, 2020.
- Brett E.Ruffo, Anorectal abscess, Chapter 13,pg372, Colorectal Surgery 2015 Corman
- Buchanan G, Halligan S, Bartram CL, et al. Clinical examination, endosonography, and MR imaging in preoperative assessment of fistula in ano: Radiology 2004, 233(30):674–81.
- de Miguel Criado J, del Salto LG, Rivas PF, del Hoyo LF, Velasco LG, de las Vacas MI, Marco Sanz AG, Paradela MM, Moreno EF. MR imaging evaluation of perianal fistulas: spectrum of imaging features. Radiographics. 2012 Jan-Feb; 32(1):175–94. Doi: 10.1148/rg.321115040. PMID: 22236900. [PubMed]
- Eisenhammer, S. (1966). The anorectal fistulous abscess and fistula. Diseases of the Colon & Rectum, 9(2), 91–106.
- Eisenhammer S. The final evaluation and classification of the surgical treatment of the primary anorectal cryptoglandular intermuscular (inter-sphincteric) fistulous abscess and fistula. Dis Colon Rectum. 1978 May-Jun;21(4):237–54. Doi 10.1007/BF02586698. PMID: 657933.
- EISENHAMMER S. The internal anal sphincter; its surgical importance. S Afr Med J. 1953 Mar 28;27(13):266–70. PMID: 13076663.
- EISENHAMMER S. The internal anal sphincter and the anorectal abscess. Surg Gynecol Obstet. 1956 Oct;103(4):501-6. PMID: 13360660.
- Garg P, Kaur B, Yagnik VD, & Dawka, S. (2021). A New Anatomical Pathway of Spread of Pus/Sepsis in Anal Fistulas Discovered on MRI and Its Clinical Implications. Clinical and experimental gastroenterology, 397–404.
- Goligher JC, Ellis M, Pissidis AG. A critique of anal glandular infection in the etiology and treatment of idiopathic anorectal abscesses and fistulas. Br J Surg. 1967 Dec;54(12):977-83. doi: 10.1002/bjs.1800541202. PMID: 6066322.[PubMed].
- Hanley PH. Reflections on anorectal abscess fistula: 1984. Dis Colon Rectum. 1985 Jul;28(7):528–33. doi: 10.1007/BF02554105. PMID: 3893948.[PubMed].
- Herand Abcarian. Classification and management strategies Anal Fistula. Anal fistula surgery. Springer DOI 10.1007/978-1-4614-9014-2_5.Springer Science+Business Media, New York 2014.
- Lunniss PJ. (1994). Aspects of fistula-in-ano. University of London, University College London (United Kingdom). [Google Scholar]
- ML Prasad, DR Read, and H. Abcarian, "Supralevator abscess: diagnosis and treatment," Diseases of the Colon and Rectum, vol. 24, no. 6, pp. 456–61, 1981. View at:[Google Scholar]
- Mappes HJ, & Farthmann EH. (2001). Anal abscess and fistula. In Surgical Treatment: Evidence-Based and Problem-Oriented. Zuckschwerdt.
- MORGAN CN. The surgical anatomy of the ischiorectal space. Proc R Soc Med. 1949 Mar;42(3):189–200. PMID: 18126986; PMCID: PMC2081231.
- Murad-Regadas SM, Dealcanfreitas ID, Oliveira MTCCD, Pessoa Morano D, Regadas FSP, Rodrigues LV, & Regadas Filho, FSP. (2015). Anatomical characteristics of anal fistula evaluated by three-dimensional anorectal ultrasonography: is there a correlation with Goodsall's theory? Journal of Coloproctology (Rio de Janeiro), 35, 8389 [Google Scholar]
- Practice parameters for the management of perianal abscess and fistula-in-ano. Steele SR, Kumar R, Feingold DL, Rafferty JL, Buie WD, Standards Practice Task Force of the American Society of Colon and Rectal Surgeons. Dis Colon Rectum. 2011 Dec; 54(12):1465–74. [PubMed] [Ref list]
- Sanyal S, Khan F, Ramachandra P. Successful management of a recurrent supralevator abscess: a case report. Case Rep Surg. 2012;2012:871639. Doi: 10.1155/2012/871639. Epub 2012 May 7. PMID: 22649747; PMCID: PMC3357932.
- Sharma A, Yadav P, Sahu M. et al. Current imaging techniques for evaluation of fistula in ano: a review. Egypt J Radiol Nucl Med 51, 130 (2020).
- Sigmon DF, Emmanuel B, Tuma F. Perianal Abscess. 2021 Jun 29. In: Stat Pearls [Internet]. Treasure Island (FL): Stat Pearls Publishing; 2021 Jan. PMID: 29083652. [PubMed]
- Treasure Island (FL): Stat Pearls Publishing; 2021 Jan. PMID: 32809492. [PubMed]

CHAPTER 7

Anatomy of Pudendal Nerve

PUDENDAL NERVE

The Latin term *pudenda* means 'external genitals'. Each side of the perineum has pudendal nerve. It provides sensation and motor function to the perineum and the external genitalia. The pelvic region sends sensory signals to the brain via the pudendal nerve. Seventy percent of the fibres in the pudendal nerve are somatic (20% are motor and 50% are sensory), and 30% are autonomic. The nerves carry sensations to the penis and clitoris, vaginal vestibule, the lower one-fifth of the vaginal canal, labia minora, scrotum and the labia majora's posterior aspects. It regulates the somatic muscles that cause penile and clitoral erection and assists in male ejaculation.

Origin: The pudendal nerve originates from the sacral plexus, specifically S2–S4.

Course: It reaches the pelvic cavity via the greater sciatic foramen, passes the sacrospinous ligament, and then re-enters the pelvis by the smaller sciatic foramen. Before reaching its target regions, the pudendal nerve follows the ischial spine and the pudendal canal, also called Alcock's canal. Alcock's canal is a bony passageway that connects the greater sciatic foramen to the ischial spine and is situated in the pelvic area. It houses the pudendal nerve, pudendal vessels, and other minor nerves (Table 7.1 and Fig. 7.1).

TABLE 7.1: NERVE SUPPLY OF BRANCHES OF THE PUDENDAL NERVE AT A GLANCE

Inferior rectal branch	*Perineal branch (Deep)*	*Perineal branch (Superficial)*	*Dorsal branch*
Sensory innervation to • Posterior vulvar region • Caudal third of the rectum • Skin of the anal circumference	**Sensory innervation to** • Lower third of the vagina and urethra	**Sensory innervation to** • Labia majora • Labia minora • Posterior portion of perianal skin	**Sensory innervation to** • Corpus cavernosum recti, which has erectile tissue. • Crus of penis • Skin of clitoris • Skin over the dorsolateral aspect of the foreskin • Glans
Motor • Levator ani muscle	**Motor** • External anal sphincter • Deep transverse and superficial perineal muscle • Bulbospongiosus • Ischiocavernosus • Urethral sphincter • External anal sphincter	**Motor** • External anal sphincter • Levator ani	**Motor** • Muscle involved in erection (Bulbospongiosus and ischiocavernosus)
Autonomic Awareness of the need to defecate	**Autonomic** Awareness of the sensation to urinate		**Autonomic** Erectile initiation and maintenance

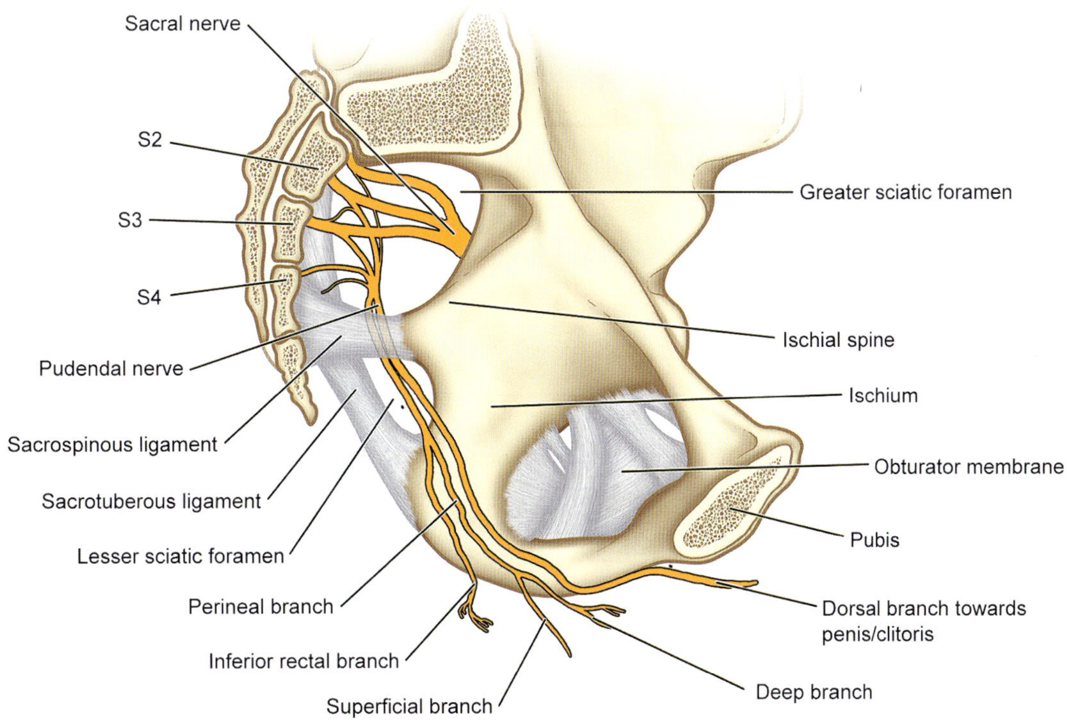

Fig. 7.1: Course of pudendal nerve

Branches of Pudendal Nerve

As it reaches the perineum, the pudendal nerve divides into 3 branches.

a. ***Inferior rectal nerve (IRN):*** Supplies the EAS, levator ani, the skin of the anus, and the lower rectal mucosa. It exits the pudendal canal, travels through the ischioanal fossa's fat, and reaches the lateral aspect of the anal canal.

   Function

   - Gives sensory supply to the inferior portion of the anal canal and the circumanal skin.
   - Provides motor supply to the EAS

b. ***Perineal nerve:*** It is pudendal nerve's largest branch. It supplies the urogenital diaphragm (Fig. 7.2A and B). It bifurcates into:

   A deep (muscular) branch that supplies

   - The muscles of the urogenital triangle
   - The external urethral sphincter
   - Levator ani
   - The anterior parts of the EAS (Fig. 7.2B)

   A superficial (cutaneous) branch that supplies:

   - The posterior scrotal area in males (Fig. 7.2A)
   - The labia minora and majora, vaginal vestibule, lower one-fifth of the vaginal canal in females

   It provides sensation to the scrotum in males and the labia in females

c. ***Dorsal nerve:*** Provides sensation to the clitoris and the penis (Fig. 7.2A).

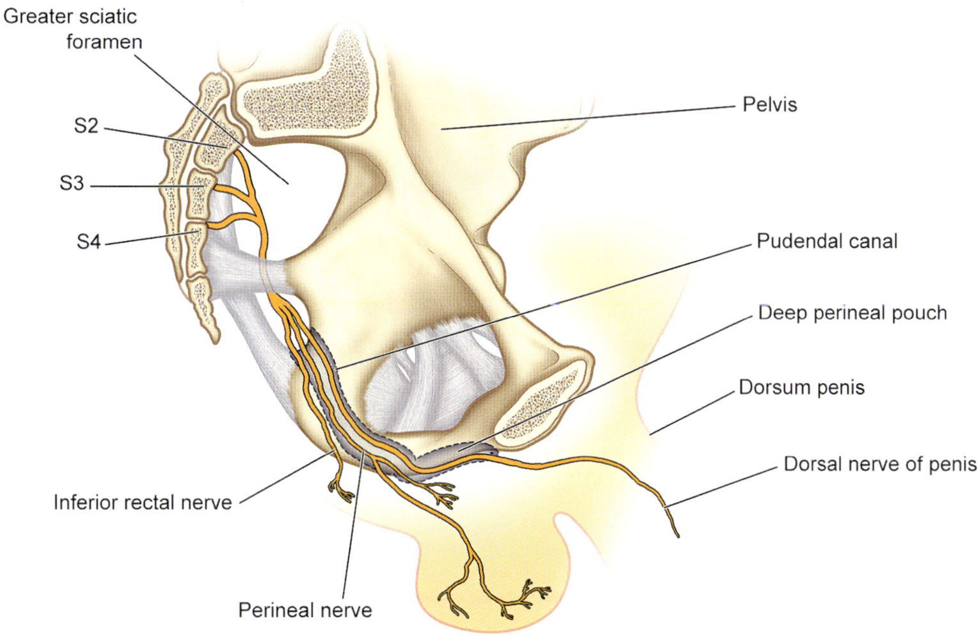

Fig. 7.2A: Branches of pudendal nerve in male perineum

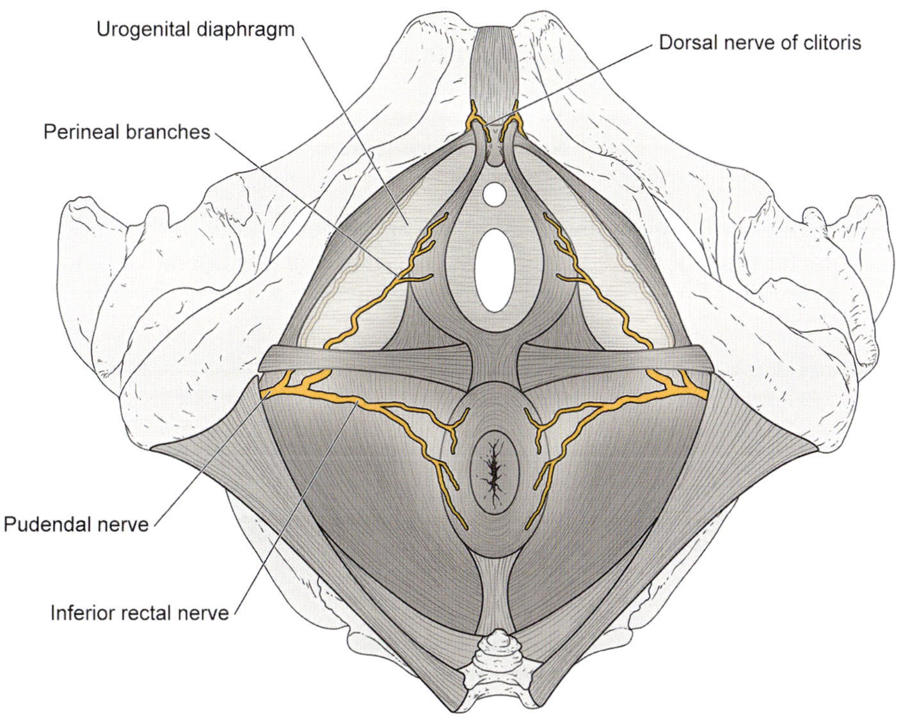

Fig. 7.2B: Perianal branches

Depth of Pudendal Nerve

The depth of the pudendal nerve may vary. However, it is commonly found 2–5 cm below the surface of the perineum and is located between the anal orifice and the scrotum or the vulva.

Pudendal Nerve Entrapment

Pudendal nerve entrapment is characterized by pudendal nerve compression, causing neuralgia along the path of the affected nerve's distribution.

The condition can be classified into different types on the basis of the location of entrapment:

- *Type I:* Entrapment is in the sciatic notch at the level of the piriformis muscle (Fig. 7.3).
- *Type II:* Entrapment is at the level of the sacrotuberous ligament as well as the ischial spine.
- *Type III:* Entrapment is within the Alcock's canal.
  - *Type IIIa:* Compression of the obturator internus muscle alone.
  - *Type IIIb:* Compression of both obturator internus and piriformis muscles.
- *Type IV:* Entrapment of the pudendal nerve's distal branches.

Pudendal Neuralgia

- It is a severe neuropathy that affects the pudendal nerve in its distribution region. It is characterized by numbness, discomfort or tingling in the vagina, vulva , glans penis, and scrotum. Pudendal nerve entrapment, mechanical injury, viral infection, and immunologic reactions are some of the reasons for pudendal neuralgia.
- Unilateral pudendal neuropathy can cause fecal incontinence.

Surgical Significance

Pudendal Nerve Block

The pudendal nerve block can be given by injecting an anaesthetic agent in the pudendal nerve. The block helps to perform anorectal surgical procedures and also in reducing postoperative pain.

Conclusion

A surgeon should be familiar with the anatomy and the course of pudendal nerve for giving pudendal nerve block and to understand the clinical conditions associated with pudendal neuropathy and pudendal nerve entrapment syndrome. The block is effective in reducing the postoperative VAS score remarkably.

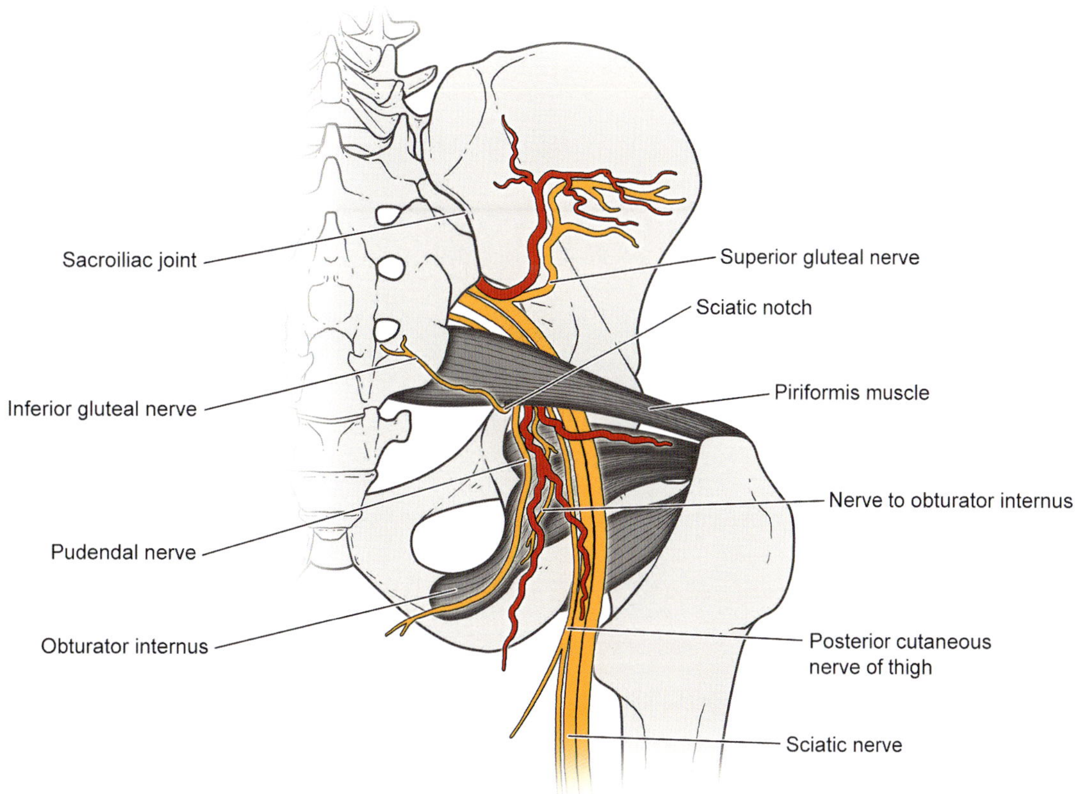

Fig. 7.3: Type 1 pudendal nerve entrapment at the piriformis level

Further Reading

- Alexis MP. Schizas, Andrew B. Williams,1 - Anorectal investigation, Editor(s): Robin K.S. Phillips, Sue Clark, Colorectal Surgery (Fifth Edition), W.B. Saunders,2014, Pages 1–16, ISBN 9780702049651,https://doi.org/10.1016/B978-0-7020-4965-1.00001-9
- Colebunders B, Matthew MK, Broer N, Persing JA, Dellon AL. Benjamin Alcock and the pudendal canal. J Reconstr Microsurg. 2011 Jul;27(6):349–54. doi: 10.1055/s-0031-1278705. Epub 2011 May 27. Erratum in: J Reconstr Microsurg. 2012 Oct;28(8):571. Broerm, Niclas [corrected to Broer, Niclas]. PMID: 21623563.
- Kinter KJ, Newton BW. Anatomy, Abdomen, and Pelvis, Pudendal Nerve. [Updated 2023 Feb 10]. In: StatPearls [Internet]. Treasure Island (FL): StatPearls Publishing; 2023 Jan. Available from: https://www.ncbi.nlm.nih.gov/books/NBK554736/
- Leslie SW, Antolak S, Feloney MP, et al. Pudendal Neuralgia. [Updated 2022 Nov 28]. In: StatPearls [Internet]. Treasure Island (FL): StatPearls Publishing; 2023 Jan. Available from: https://www.ncbi.nlm.nih.gov/books/NBK562246/
- Oelhafen K, Shayota BJ, Muhleman M, Klaassen Z, Tubbs RS, Loukas M. Benjamin Alcock (1801-?) and his canal. Clin Anat. 2013 Sep;26(6):662–6. doi: 10.1002/ca.22080. Epub 2012 Apr 9. PMID: 22488487.
- The Pudendal Nerve https://teachmeanatomy.info/pelvis/other/pudendal-nerve/
- Weech D, Ameer MA, Ashurst JV. Anatomy, Abdomen and Pelvis, Penis Dorsal Nerve. [Updated 2022 Aug 8]. In: StatPearls [Internet]. Treasure Island (FL): StatPearls Publishing; 2023 Jan. Available from: https://www.ncbi.nlm.nih.gov/books/NBK525966/